The Essential Dog Owner's Manual for CCL Injury

WHAT TO DO BEFORE, DURING & AFTER SURGERY

Carla J. Spinelli

Foreword by Catherine Popovitch, DVM, DACVS, DECVS

D1532276

This book is dedicated to Catherine A. Popovitch, DVM, DACVS, DECVS. Thank you for your sound advice, surgical expertise and care of my beloved pet.

Thanks to you, my dog is whole again and loving life.

A special thank you to Lisa Byrne. Your edits, patience and suggestions made a world of difference.

To my dog, Vinny, a kiss and a pat on the head for being a brave little guy and making it through two major orthopedic surgeries. Thank you for being patient with me and for being a good teacher so we can help other pet owners and their dogs.

Table of Contents

Foreword

Our pets are such an important part of our life and family. When they're injured, we want the best care possible for them. We seek advice from veterinarians. We may even do some internet research. However, the medical information that we're presented with can often be overwhelming and confusing.

Damage to the cranial cruciate ligament is by far the most common canine orthopedic injury. Having gone through the surgery (twice) with her dog Vinny, Carla Spinelli has put her experience and insights into this very helpful book. She discusses the pre-surgery decision making process then guides you through the post-operative recovery process. This book is a valuable resource for anyone whose beloved pet requires cruciate surgery.

- Catherine A. Popovitch, DVM, DACVS, DECVS

Introduction – Why I Wrote This Book

I was overwhelmed with stress, confusion and worry in deciding which path I'd take to help my dog recover from his torn CCL (cranial cruciate ligament). Every spare minute, I'd jump on the Internet to research. From blogs and articles to forums and YouTube videos, I spent countless hours trying to learn everything I could.

I wrote this book so you wouldn't have to do what I did – spend exorbitant amounts of time fretting over what to do and never feeling convinced about which path to take. I've outlined the material to cut to the chase. It's valuable for anyone whose dog has a cruciate ligament injury that may or may not require surgery. My goal is to calm you down and help you feel less afraid of the process.

You'll find my additional CCL related information below. Join, read and listen. And whatever you do – don't worry. You CAN rock the recovery!

Facebook: https://www.facebook.com/groups/CCLsurgery/
Podcast: https://anchor.fm/runagainrover
Web: www.RunAgainRover.com
Instagram: @RunAgainRover

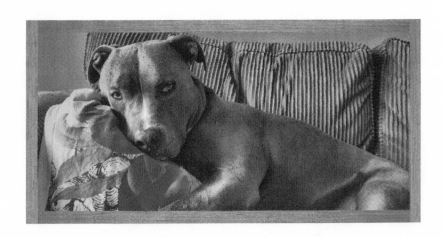

Why You Should Read This Book

There's so much information out there, but the first challenge is knowing where to look. Considering the endless blogs, websites and videos, there's lots of valuable information and just as much that's incorrect. This is the stuff that gets people and their pets into trouble.

Then you have to culminate everything you've learned to come up with a solid plan of action and how you'll carry out those actions. You'll ask yourself:

"Can I do this myself or will I need help?"
"How much money am I willing to spend?"
"If my dog needs surgery, which technique is best?"
"Will I need to take time off from work?"

I had a difficult time finding one book or website that covered the entire process including before, during and after knee surgery. Most of the material explained various surgical options or laid out how to do post-op rehabilitation, but what about everything in between?

Culling information was an arduous task and inspired me to make it easier for others. I brought the information together and put it into one resource. Relax - the hard part is done.

You can trust what I've written because nothing beats real-life experience. My dog, Vinny, injured both of his CCL's. He had two TPLO's that were a mere eight-months apart.

Going through the experience twice made me feel more at ease the second time around. There were surprising differences in his healing, ability to get around after surgery and reactions to medications. I'll share everything I learned from both procedures.

I wrote this book for you, the one about to embark into a brave new world with the hope of helping your dog live an enjoyable, robust life. Even if you intend to begin with conservative management and may consider surgery in the future, this material will help you get prepared, informed and more at ease with what lies ahead.

To make reading simpler, I refer to dogs using male pronouns only.

I assured Vinny this book could be his claim to fame, so throughout you will find pictures of him. Sometimes they'll relate to the chapter material, and sometimes they won't. Either way, we think you'll enjoy seeing them!

Please take a moment to post a book review on Amazon. It will help others know that what you read was valuable. Here's the link: https://amzn.to/2SbIYSH

Thank you.

Researching Caused Confusion

I believed that the more research I did, the more prepared and confident I'd be about whatever decision I made. But that didn't happen. The more I read, the more confused and nervous I became.

There are a lot of strong and differing opinions about the best ways treat torn CCL's. For some people it's an easy decision – they simply go with their vet's recommendations. Others might need to research and weigh the pros and cons between non-invasive versus surgical options. The factors that go into moving forward with surgery are more complex than you might think.

Here are some factors to consider.

- Your financial investment toward surgery and supplies
- Your physical ability and strength
- Whether you'll have help in caring for your dog
- Your dog's age and physical condition
- The amount of time you have to give to his recuperation
- Your ability to have a flexible schedule
- The layout of your house
- Your willingness to live "rough" for some time
- Making temporary house and yard modifications

You see? It's not only about how much the surgery costs. It's about considering the challenges you'll face before, during and after the procedure.

Trying to avoid surgery, I spent a month managing my dog conservatively believing he would heal. I decreased and modified his usual activities.

Conservative management consists of any nonsurgical treatment of injuries including: physical therapy, hydrotherapy, cold laser treatments, chiropractic adjustments, acupuncture, massage, nutrition, a stifle brace, non-steroidal anti-inflammatory drugs (NSAIDS), medicinal herbs and other supplements, weight loss for overweight dogs and other noninvasive treatments.

Making the Decision to Have Surgery

I gave the non-surgical route an honest try. When I saw that he wasn't progressing the way I hoped he would, I knew I needed to move forward. I revisited the research I had done previously and attempted to read it in a different vein.

I combed through articles describing various surgical procedures: Lateral Suture Technique (extracapsular lateral suture stabilization), Tightrope repair, TPLO, CBLO and TTA. I decided on lateral suture because it didn't involve cutting through bone (osteotomy) and was therefore less invasive than the other options. I was relieved to have made the decision.

I scheduled the first veterinary consult and ran into my first roadblock. The lateral suture technique, the one I had my heart set on, is most suitable for lighter weight, less active dogs. My dog is an 80-pound bundle of muscle and exuberant energy. Would the lateral suture hold up over time or would he need a second stronger repair (surgical revision) if the first one didn't work? I struggled with whether it was the right procedure for him. I didn't want him to suffer through two painful surgeries. And I certainly didn't want to pay for multiple procedures.

Regarding expense: CCL surgeries are costly, especially if you don't have pet insurance. I didn't have it then and still don't. There are factors to consider besides the cost of surgery itself.

Consultation fees can run between $75 and $150 each. Add to that the cost for additional items such as a harness or sling to lift your dog and help him walk, supplements, prescription medications, a heated dog mat, an orthopedic dog bed, an exercise pen, and other helpers for managing your dog's comfort.

If you decide on surgery, options besides paying out of pocket include Care Credit. They have flexible plans that can be paid back over time. You could use social media to ask for help from family and friends. Setting up a GoFundMe page is a way for people to offer donations to help for surgery and supplies. There are fundraising companies such as Bonfire and Ink to the People where you can create and sell a T-shirt with your dog's pic on it. For more fun ideas, please check out my fundraising post on my site at www.RunAgainRover.com.

There's a section toward the end of this book that lists the items I purchased for my dog. You don't need to take notes about products as I mention them. At the end of the book, you'll see my Amazon Affiliate store link where you can see or purchase the items I used to help Vinny before, during and after surgery. If you purchase products through my affiliate link I receive a small commission, maybe enough to buy myself a fancy-schmancy latté or two.

Whether you choose conservative management or surgery, each has advantages and drawbacks. And when you think about it, isn't that the way it goes with many of the choices we have to consider? This is no different. There's no miracle solution or quick fix.

Vinny's Story

This is my pit bull, Vinny. He's a stubborn, energetic, strong and loving boy who loves to chase birds and animals in his yard. That's what started the ordeal with his knee. He overzealously chased a skunk and wound up being not only super stinky but walked away with a sore left knee. He hobbled around and was what veterinarians refer to as "three-legged lame".

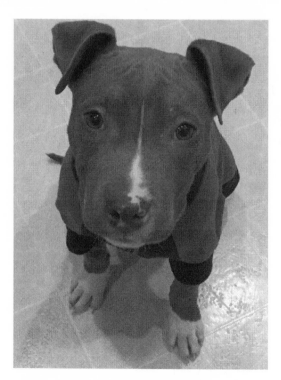

Some days were better than others. At times he limped by not putting full weight on his injured leg or he hopped on three legs.

As time progressed so did the limping, a sign that pain was worsening. Despite that, there were times when he'd run and jump as though his knee was perfectly healthy. Allowing him to do that was a big mistake, which I'll address later.

A month or so after injuring his left knee he began limping on the right hind leg. Ugh! I read about how common it was that once one side tears, the other could too.

Vinny exhibited every symptom I read about. Rather than walking normally, he'd do occasional bunny hops with both back legs. Instead of sitting with just the injured left leg straight out or winged-out to the side, both hind legs were straight. When he stood to eat or when he wanted to walk in the opposite direction, he shifted the majority of his body weight toward the front of his body.

His upper body became contracted. It was visible when standing and walking, and I felt the muscle tightness when I massaged him. Everything happened so fast; it was as though a new symptom appeared each day. I suppose it was the kick in the butt that I needed to schedule surgery. It was difficult to see him struggle. I felt like a failure, even though I knew there was never any promise that conservative therapies would help. I felt a lot of guilt for letting the injury go on for so long and not giving in to surgery sooner.

I moved to the next phase, which was to get surgical consults. As soon as I made the decision I learned everything I could about the canine stifle (knee) joint and the best surgical methods of dealing with CCL injury. Information about the consultations is included in an upcoming chapter.

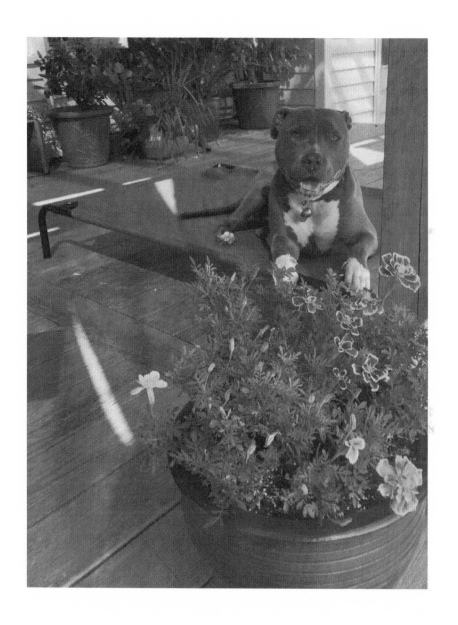

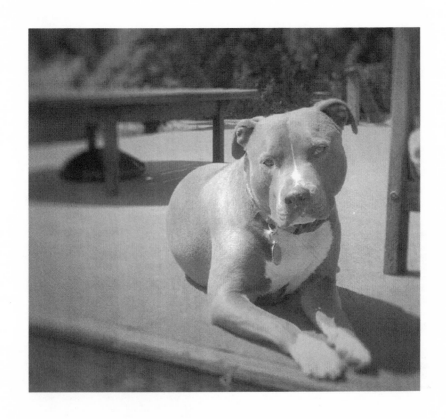

Why the CCL Tears

These anatomical terms might be new to you, so I'll review them to help you gain an understanding of structures located in the leg and knee.

- Femur = thigh bone
- Tibia = shin bone
- Stifle = knee joint
- Hock = ankle joint
- Tibial plateau = the top of the tibia

Surprisingly, canine and human knees are quite similar! Like humans, dogs have ligaments in their knee to stabilize the joint as it moves. There are two stabilizing ligaments in each leg.

The human ligaments are called the Anterior Cruciate Ligament (ACL) and the Posterior Cruciate Ligament (PCL).

In dogs, the Caudal Cruciate Ligament is the equivalent to the human PCL. The other is the Cranial Cruciate Ligament, which is like the human ACL. This is the one that tears most often in dogs. Its major job is to prevent anterior shifting (tibial thrust) of the tibia as the dog bears weight. In the literature, abbreviations CCL, CrCL and ACL are used synonymously. In this book, I'll use the CCL abbreviation.

There's an excellent YouTube video by a Board-Certified veterinary surgeon, Dr. Michael Bauer. He explains in four minutes why so many dogs tear their CCLs/ACLs.

He's a fantastic educator and teaches things in ways that are easy-to-understand. Type this URL into your web browser to see his video: https://bit.ly/2y8B2Gz

When you look at your dog from the side as he stands you'll see a slight bend at the knee. Because of this slightly flexed position, when your dog is standing, walking, running and jumping, the CCL has significant tension placed on it. This is especially true when your dog runs and jumps. The constant tension on the CCL is one reason for its susceptibility to injury and why CCL tear is the most common orthopedic injury and the leading cause of hind leg lameness in dogs.

When a dog is active, there's a small amount of shifting or shearing force between the two major leg bones, the larger femur (top of the leg) and the smaller tibia (bottom of the leg). Certain breeds have knee anatomy (steep tibial angle) that predisposes the femur to slide caudally (toward the back or tail end of the dog's body) and rub on the back of the tibia, resulting in inflammation and pain.

No matter how it happens, CCL tears result in pain and inflammation. This is why most dogs with this injury hesitate to put weight on the leg. If they do, they barely touch the paw to the ground. The mere act of sitting comfortably with a torn CCL becomes painful, which is why dogs sit bearing more weight on the uninjured side with the injured leg winging out to the side.

Here's how to envision the CCL. Think of a durable cable that's attached to something from above and below. If we cut halfway through the center (this represents a partial CCL tear), it frays and loses tensile strength. It stretches farther than it should. The parts above and below its connection points (the femur and tibia) have lost their strong anchor and can excessively shear or shift. A partially torn CCL can withstand minor forces. But with successive loading it continues to break down.

In the case of a full thickness tear of the CCL, the acute force or chronic degradation was significant enough to sever the ligament the entire way through. When that happens, the knee is highly unstable.

When vets perform the Drawer Test and the Tibial Compression test, they're assessing whether and to what degree the CCL allows the tibia to shift forward relative to the femur. Here are the most common reasons for CCL tears:

- An acute tear related to an injury (slip, fall, running...)
- Overweight dogs have continual biomechanical stress in their knees.
- There could be a hormonal connection related to premature spaying.
- Dogs that are typically sedentary who have episodes of physical overexertion (a lazy dog who is taken on a hike)
- Certain breeds are more prone to CCL injury than others because of their physical confirmation and steep tibial plateau angles.

While all of these are worth consideration, the majority of studies focus on wear and tear stress in the ligament making it the most often cited reason for CCL injury.

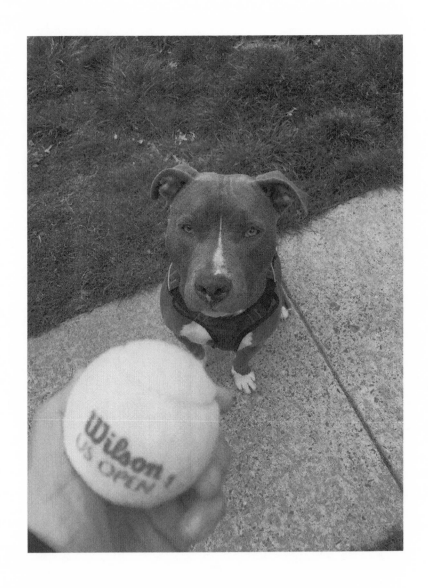

Is My Dog Too Old for Surgery?

My dog was still young when he hurt himself. I wanted him to be able to enjoy life. I knew that if conservative care didn't work, surgery was inevitable. Knowing he was healthy and young made the decision to move forward with surgery a bit easier to make.

For an older dog here are some details to review with the surgeon: underlying health conditions, activity level prior to injury, and medications or supplements you give him. Older dogs might need blood tests or other diagnostic studies before undergoing surgery. Be sure to ask about this ahead of time.

Not every older dog will be content lying around all day because his knee hurts. Think about people for a moment. There are active older adults who have more energy than younger people I know! I'm sure they wouldn't succumb to resting all day because of knee pain. Surgical repair allows people of all ages to resume activities that bring them joy. The same holds true for our pets.

Consider the years your dog has left to live. If he's happy lounging and doesn't care about romping around or taking long walks, perhaps conservative care options are best. But if your dog loves playing fetch, hiking, swimming or chasing birds and squirrels, surgery should be considered.

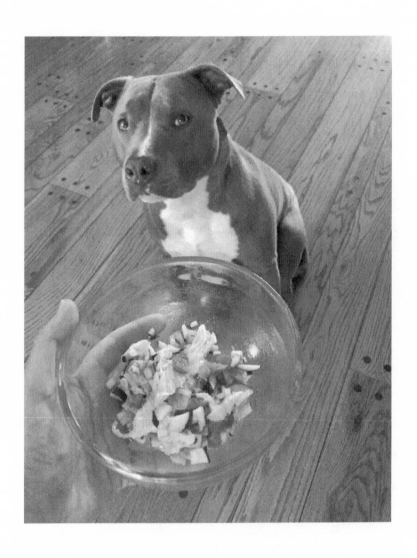

Activities That Injure the CCL

Think about how your dog's back legs look just before he or she jumps. His bottom lowers toward the ground a bit, his hind legs bend at the knee, and then a forceful straightening happens from the back legs that propel movement upward.

You can mimic the movement yourself by standing up, slightly squatting down and jumping upward. It's that same bending to straightening mechanism that loads and creates a lot of force inside your dog's knee joint.

That stated, don't allow your dog to:

- run up or down stairs
- jump on or off furniture
- roughhouse with people or other pets
- be off-leash while outside
- play with or chase other pets, birds or wild animals

It's difficult to adhere to activity restriction, and you might feel guilt for not allowing him to do things that dogs inherently do. Sure, he'll be bored, but don't let it weaken you into allowing him to run in the yard thinking it will do him some good. That was one of the mistakes I repeatedly made.

Excessive motion in an injured knee inhibits healing, increases pain and limping and often contributes to tearing the CCL in the opposite leg.

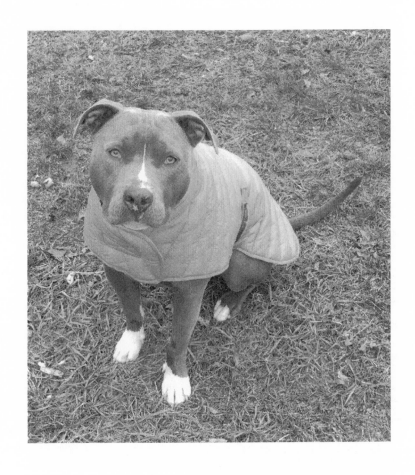

Does Your Dog Have Arthritis?

The quick answer to this is, "Yes". It's highly likely that with the torn CCL there's also some arthritis.

Arthritis forms when there's joint dysfunction. With a torn CCL the joint isn't as stable as it used to be. Bones aren't anchored strongly and therefore move excessively. The joint gets inflamed, the space between the bones decreases, cartilage thins and bone spurs form. That's what arthritis is. Also known as osteoarthritis, it's the body's normal, unstoppable and natural attempt at repairing itself.

With every injury, the body goes into healing mode. Edema (swelling) infiltrates the injured area. Bone cells, called osteoblasts, are called in to repair bones. Slowly, they build spur-like projections. These extra bone growths, called osteophytes, put pressure on adjacent tissues such as cartilage, other bones, nerves, muscles, ligaments and connective tissue. This results in decreased range of motion and pain.

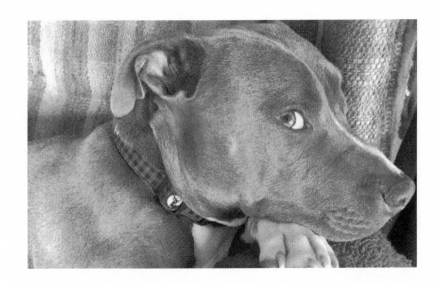

Managing Your Dog's Weight

Your dog isn't as active as he was before his knee injury. Since he's not expending as much energy, consider slightly decreasing food portions. Overweight dogs have extra stress on their knees so it's essential to get an overweight dog leaner. This should happen slowly. Rapid weight loss is unhealthy and potentially dangerous. Helping him lose weight could be as simple as not feeding table scraps or decreasing the number of treats he gets.

If you're attempting to decrease his weight, please get professional help to learn how many calories are needed to properly nourish your pet.

You might consider gradually switching to a better-quality food. There is much debate about food brands. Some veterinarians and pet parents believe that foods containing corn, soy, rice and animal byproducts brand kibble are healthy, but many people disagree.

Just as there are veterinarians who achieved a higher level of training to be able to do orthopedic surgeries, there are doctors who specialize in pet nutrition. If you're interested in learning more about which food is healthiest for your pet/s, I recommend getting the information from a specialist.

No matter which food brand you decide on, switching brands abruptly can cause stomach upset. It's important to transition from one food to another by slowly adding small amounts of the new food to the old one. Eventually, the entire serving will be the new food.

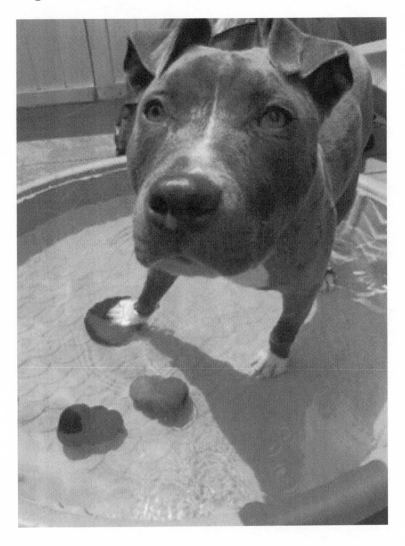

Pain Serves a Purpose

Pain is a signal that reminds us (and our pets) that there's a problem. Here's a human example of how pain protects us. Let's say you're outside doing yard work. Bending, twisting and lifting leaves you with back pain. The next day the pain worsens.

Think of what would happen if we injured ourselves and there wasn't a pain signal to remind us that there was a problem. We'd continue to do more bending, lifting or exercising and the injury could worsen. This is the reason that some people believe that using medication to get rid of pain isn't the best option. Pain medication can mask pain to the point that your dog runs and jumps, which you know isn't good for his injured knee.

There's a fine line between allowing some pain versus too much. If your dog hasn't had surgery, when should you consider asking the vet for medication to decrease pain and inflammation?

- When your pet has difficulty getting up from sitting or lying
- When your dog shows signs of distress such as quivering, shaking, panting, snapping or biting
- When limping increases
- If you notice that both back legs are hurting. Evidence of this is lifting either hind paw off the ground as he stands, sitting with the back legs winged-out or straight rather than evenly tucked beneath the body, limping with either back leg
- If he whimpers, whines or yelps with movement

• If the hind leg or paw feels warmer or appears swollen compared to the uninjured leg

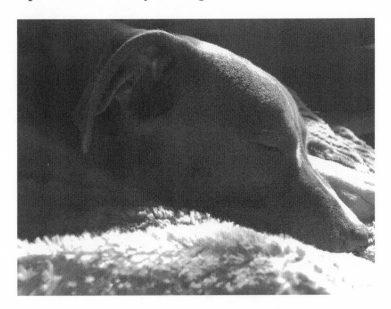

Conservative Management 101

When humans injure their ACL, an orthopedist usually begins by recommending a non-surgical approach called conservative management. This might include medications, physical therapy, ice pack or heating pad application, rest and avoiding activities that load the knee joint with pressure. This approach can also be applied to your dog.

I began treating Vinny's CCL injury conservatively because I wanted to avoid surgery.

The first month after his injury. I modified the size of the yard to control his running freedom. I staked out and fenced in a smaller section so he couldn't run as fast or as far. I allowed him to go out to do his business without being leashed. At times he played with toys or jogged around to patrol his new smaller yard. Although making the outside area smaller was an excellent move, allowing him to run off leash was not. I'll address this in a section called "My Mistakes".

Surgery isn't the answer for every dog. If your dog isn't in excruciating pain, you could try conservative management and rest. At the very least it could provide you with more definitive answers as to whether surgery is necessary or not. Although I eventually chose TPLO for Vinny, I don't regret having tried conservative methods first.

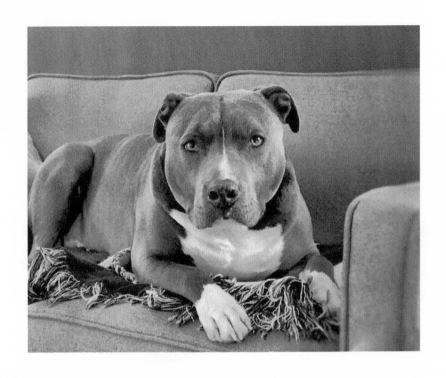

Supplements & Other Pre-Surgery Purchases

I purchased an assortment of items to help Vinny before and after surgery. These are by no means required.

The products are available in my Amazon Affiliate store at www.RunAgainRover.com.

If surgery is scheduled, I highly recommend that you get prepared before your dog returns home from the hospital by stocking up on the things you'll need. Set yourself up for success beforehand so you're not scrambling around after he's home from surgery. You'll be less anxious and your pup will be happier with you nearby.

Heated Mat

One of the first things I purchased was a heated mat for him to lie on. He accepted this better than when I tried putting a heating pad on his leg. Heat application is especially helpful during cold or damp weather. When he lies on the heated mat he's less stiff and has an easier time standing up from a lying position compared to when he lies on a cold, drafty floor. Having the heated mat will be especially helpful during cold weather seasons and later in life, when joints and muscles tend to stiffen.

If you use a heating pad to soothe his knee, place a layer or two of a dish towel (not a paper towel) between his body and the heating pad. The towel will help the leg to not get overly hot. After 10 minutes, remove the heating pad and allow a half hour or more before you reapply it. You don't want to keep the area overly warm for extended periods of time.

Supplements

When Vinny first hurt his knee, he never cried out in pain or whimpered. Although I couldn't see any swelling, I knew it was deep inside, so my conservative treatment plan included these anti-inflammatory supplements:

- Turmeric. It's absorbed best when given with fat, such as with an Omega-3 supplement. Piperine, in black pepper, increases the bioavailability of turmeric.
- Omega-3 fatty acids from sardines and anchovies. There's less mercury, a harmful neurotoxin, found in smaller fish versus larger ones like salmon
- Cosequin, a glucosamine and chondroitin supplement
- Yucca root extract
- Glycoflex Stage 3 glucosamine chewy supplements
- Standard Process Ligaplex II supplement
- Perna canine chew treats

I staggered giving him the supplements so his tummy wouldn't get upset from getting them all at once. I supplemented for a month and didn't notice a major difference. The only adverse reaction was vomiting, which was caused by Cosequin. It was the culprit because it was the only supplement he was taking at that time. Do note: many dogs take Cosequin without problems. I switched to a joint supplement made for humans, also suitable for dogs, called Ligaplex II.

Car/Stair Ramp

I considered purchasing a ramp to help him get in and out of my car. I didn't end up getting one because I had help picking him up from the hospital and bringing him into the house. After surgery, he was so woozy from the anesthesia that there was no way he could have used one anyway.

Getting a ramp could be a smart decision if you take your dog for car rides, especially if you have an SUV. Even after your dog's knee heals from surgery, a ramp will facilitate getting in and out of your vehicle. With SUV's choose a longer one to avoid having your dog walk up a steep, challenging incline. Some are covered with a grass-like non-slip material and others have a sand paper type of covering. Be aware of buyer complaints that the sand paper coating peels.

Have your dog practice walking across the ramp before surgery by laying it flat on the floor. Entice him to walk on it by offering treats and praise. Then progress with the ramp going up a couple stairs or into your car. He might be reluctant to try it if his knee is painful so don't force the situation.

If you have a lot of steps to get your dog outside, a harness is a safer option. A ramp going over too many steps will be excessively steep and possibly slip and slide.

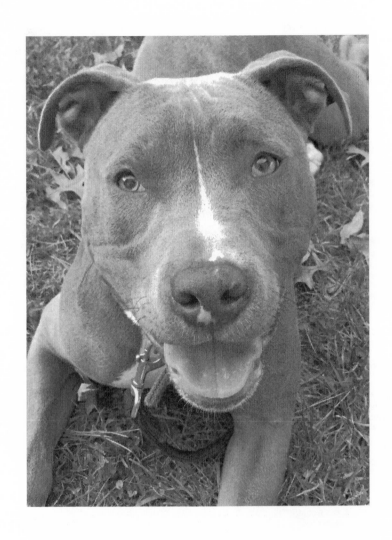

The Brace Place

Why is a brace helpful? It's designed to support your dog's knee as he walks by stabilizing and supporting the joint while limiting an excessive range of motion. Joint stabilization and limitation of movement allow scar tissue to form. You want that. Scar tissue formation is a normal part of healing in every animal. The brace doesn't do anything to fix or heal the CCL. The tear will still be there, but the scar tissue will act as an internal brace.

If your dog is going to be successful with a stifle brace, and there are no guarantees with this, it will depend on your diligence. This means it must be put on your dog first thing in the morning and removed before bed – every day. You must be sure that it fits correctly. And you need to be aware that you're in it for the long haul. For the brace to work, it needs to be worn for close to a year. Your dog might still need medications to control pain and inflammation.

When I realized that supplements alone weren't enough, I decided to try a stifle brace to support his left knee (at this point the right knee was still healthy). I did hours of research. I read lots of negative reviews and learned about design flaws that allow braces to slip, twist or rub against the already painful knee. Some of them cause chafing or skin ulcerations. With others, straps that fasten across the low back slide down whenever the dog sits or lies down.

For this reason, I *only* recommend a custom-fitted stifle brace that is made to fit from a cast of your dog's leg.

These braces are lightweight, waterproof and durable. While there are many companies that sell knee braces, I recommend these three: Hero Braces, Orthopet and My Pet's Brace.

I purchased Vinny's brace from My Pet's Brace. On our initial visit, they made a form-fitted cast of Vinny's leg, which was used to create his actual brace. We scheduled another visit to have final adjustments made so it would fit him perfectly.

The tech did an excellent job of explaining how to put it on correctly. She marked a line on the straps to ensure the tension was just right. She watched as he walked and made final adjustments. Vinny tolerated wearing it and his gait improved a bit. I followed their instructions on gradual usage, but he had his own "usage issues", which interrupted our plan.

Initially, a brace should only be worn for a couple hours per day. You'll get instructions. Wearing duration is gradually increased until eventually it's worn all day and removed at bedtime. The amount of time for stabilizing scar tissue to form is around nine months, and even though the brace stabilizes the knee you'll need to take precautions early on to keep your dog from physical overexertion.

I've got to admit, Vinny looked adorable in his shamrock green brace. Right from the start, he seemed to have an easier time walking. Your pup will need to acclimate to the sensation of wearing it, so keep a close eye on him in the beginning.

I tried being vigilant, but a few minutes of my not watching was all he needed. The little escape artist made it his mission to silently gnaw at the elastic and Velcro fasteners so he could pull the brace off. He did this on three separate occasions! That meant three separate calls to the company to order extra fasteners. They shipped via snail mail taking three-days before I received them. It made it impossible to adhere to their wearing schedule. It was just enough time for him to get used to not wearing it, so when I put the repaired brace back on, the secretive nibbling resumed.

HELPFUL HINT: When you purchase a brace, if possible order a couple sets of extra straps.

Do your research, and buy from a stifle brace company because their product and their customer service is stellar, not because they use old-school scare tactics to get you to avoid surgery and buy from them instead.

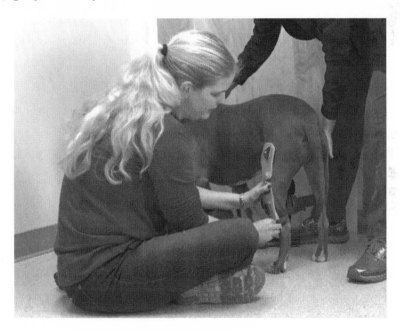

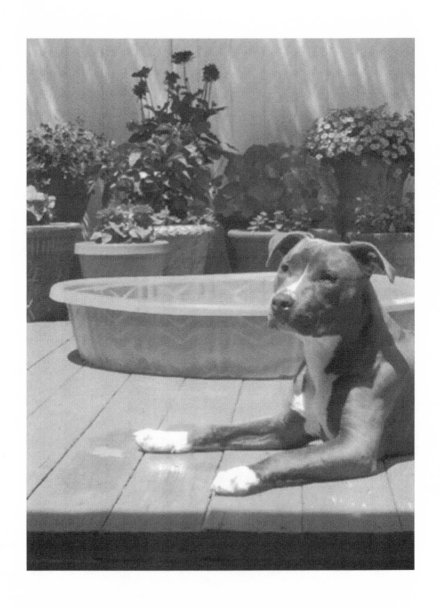

Minimizing Pain and Swelling

I brought Vinny to see his primary care veterinarian, Dr. Keith Warren. He asked lots of questions, did an examination and was the first doctor to teach me about CCL tears. He recommended that I consult with a surgeon. I asked about getting medication to help reduce swelling and pain. He prescribed Deramaxx. Vinny responded well, and the limping decreased. After two-weeks, blood work was done to show whether the drug was affecting liver and kidney enzyme levels. His levels were perfect, so Dr. Warren filled the next prescription.

The medication gave me time to decide which surgical option was most appropriate. In the meantime, I learned how to do some simple at home physical therapy techniques.

The next chapter reviews the physical therapy exercises Vinny was able to do without discomfort. You'll also learn about the ones I decided to nix from his routine.

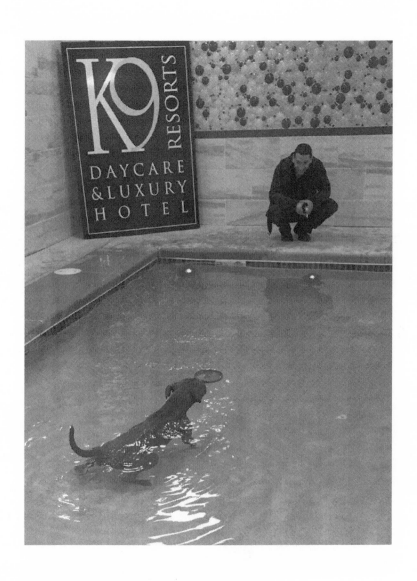

Pre-Surgery Physical Therapy Routine

When humans and animals are in pain, they avoid using the painful side. Muscles look skinny and become weak. You might notice this on your dog by comparing the "meatiness" of the healthy hind leg to the injured one. The skinniness is called "disuse atrophy". If you've ever seen a person who had a cast removed from their arm or leg, and the limb is scrawny looking - that's what disuse atrophy looks like.

Let's consider a human model for a moment: In preparation for knee replacement surgery, some orthopedists recommend physical therapy beforehand to strengthen the muscles around the joint. It's referred to as "prehab". It strengthens the muscles surrounding the joint, which helps people achieve the best possible recovery and surgical outcome.

Here's what my pre-surgery, gentle physical therapy prehab consisted of. I started by having him lie on his heated mat to warm up his legs. I massaged his shoulders and lightly massaged both back legs similar to the way human massage is done. I applied light pressure starting at the paw and moved upward toward his hip. Massage in this direction because it moves the edema from the legs back into systemic circulation. Support the undersurface of his leg at the level of the knee with one hand while you massage with the other hand.

After the massage, I did passive range of motion (PROM) exercises on his legs. This is where you manually move the leg in a natural motion, just like the movement his leg makes when he walks. These exercises are designed to maintain mobility of the knee and hip by passively moving your dog's leg for him.

Support under his knee (stifle) joint with one hand while the other hand lightly grasps around the hock (ankle) as you gently bend and straighten his leg. I never went into a full bend or full straightening. Being overzealous with passive range of motion could cause pain. You'll know if your dog is in pain because he will pull his leg back, squirm around or whimper. My dog tolerated my doing PROM therapy for three or four repetitions. As soon as he retracted his leg, I took it as his sign that it didn't feel good and that I should stop.

It was winter when I did the PT exercises so I did them indoors. There are a few things that make outdoor PT challenging. First, there are many distractions, both visual and scent related. There are squirrels, birds, people and other pets that could entice him to pull, run or jump. If it's snowy or damp outside, the ground could be lumpy, uneven or slippery. Damp fall days or wintery ones where there's snow on the ground are ones that you should consider doing PT inside if you have the space. Working inside in the warmth and on level ground will be ideal.

I chose a space in my house that was big enough to set up my "training course". If the largest space you have necessitates your dog having to go up or down a lot of stairs to access it, your best choice is to do them in a smaller area and to set up and take down each exercise after it's performed.

We began by doing big figure-8's around two kettle bells. You could use anything that's large enough to be seen by you and your pup: a gallon of water, a couple bricks or jugs of laundry detergent. Use something your dog won't be enticed to play with. I set them about nine feet apart. We did four figure-8's walking in one direction and four in the opposite direction. Don't cut tight corners; make wide turns instead. He was always leashed, and we walked slowly. I encouraged him with treats, pats on the head and lots of praise.

Next, I set up Cavaletti poles, which is like mini set-up of what an Equestrian horse jumps over. I made four of them in a row with the cross bar less than two inches off the ground. Setting the poles too high could cause knee pain as he attempts to step over them, so it's best to keep them low. Each Cavaletti pole was about four feet apart from the next. Putting them too close to one another will cause your dog to trip over them. If you only have a small room to do this in, just set up one or two poles. We did four walkovers in one direction and four in the opposite direction. He wagged his tail the entire time. He was so proud of himself!

When we finished work on our "training course", it was time for cool-down. With him lying, I draped a dishtowel over his knee and placed a small bag of frozen peas on top. This calmed any irritation caused by the activity. We did the training every other day. Overdoing PT can cause pain and limping, so my advice is to be conservative and allow a rest day in between. On the off days, I still gave him massages, which he loved! I did all four legs, his belly, chest, back and neck. It made him feel so good that he'd fall asleep every time.

Like the majority of dogs with one CCL injury, the dog relies more on the healthy hind leg. Unfortunately, this often begins the wear and tear process of the opposite CCL.

It wasn't long before I saw changes happening with his right (uninjured) leg. Consequently, I discontinued doing PT when I noticed him limping on both back legs. PT had run its course. Conservative care wasn't enough. I needed to get serious about figuring out which surgical procedure he'd have.

41

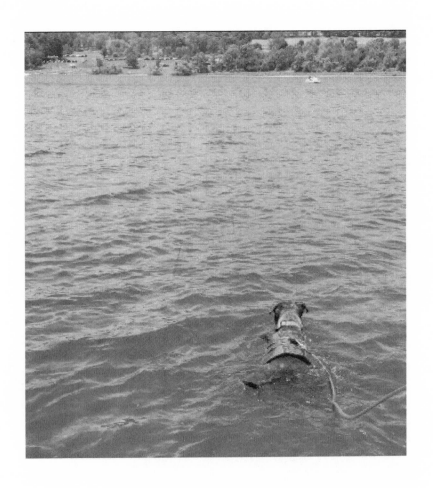

Investigating Surgical Options

I wanted Vinny to have a happy life playing and running like dogs are supposed to do. Day by day, I became increasingly convinced that surgery was necessary because his symptoms became more pronounced.

He limped more frequently, and the medication was no longer effective. His upper body and back looked and felt contracted. He had a harder time getting up from a lying position.

I read veterinary journal articles. I watched YouTube videos created by veterinarians and dog owners. I learned about the differences between CBLO, TPLO, TTA, MMP, lateral suture technique (extracapsular repair) and tightrope procedure. I wanted to be 100% certain that I had done my homework and chosen the best option.

I'll describe a human ACL tear repair and compare it to when dogs have the same tear. When a human tears an ACL (the same knee ligament as a canine CCL), an orthopedic surgeon can sometimes repair the tendon itself. This is done by re-connecting the torn pieces or by using either autograft or allograft tissue.

Autograph is when the surgeon harvests your tissue to recreate a new ACL tendon. They remove a tendon from another part of your body and use it to create a new ACL.

: is when the new ACL is gotten from a cadaver an body) and then used to make a new ACL. [ue has proven to be great options for dogs.

: comes to dogs, the majority of surgical techniques involve leaving the torn CCL alone and surgically stabilizing the bones to which the ligament attaches.

Keep in mind that with every surgical procedure there are associated risks and complications. Please ask your surgeon to review them with you.

Lateral Suture Technique & Tightrope Procedure

Initially, I preferred the lateral suture technique because it didn't completely change the biomechanics of how the knee joint moves. Rather than stabilizing with steel plates and bone screws like the CBLO, TPLO and TTA do, the lateral suture material is a durable, synthetic cord that's threaded through holes drilled through the femur and tibia. Both procedures use the cord material to control excessive movement in the stifle joint. This added stability prevents shearing forces on the torn CCL. These procedures are most appropriate for lighter weight dogs. Extra care must be taken during recovery because the suture material can fail (break) which could necessitate another surgery.

Tibial Tuberosity Advancement (TTA) & Modified Maquet Procedure (MMP)

These techniques uses a vertical bone cut through the front of the tibia to move the tibial tubercle forward. Advancing the tibial tuberosity changes the way the quadriceps (thigh) muscles pull on the front of the leg, making the quadriceps tendon act similarly to an intact cruciate ligament. This procedure uses a metal implant to maintain the space within the vertically cut tibia. The MMP uses a newer type of implant called Orthofoam. This titanium wedge is porous, allowing for bone to grow through the implant. This is said to create a strong, stable repair.

Tibial Plateau Leveling Osteotomy (TPLO)

This surgical procedure alters the dynamics of the knee by using a curved bone cut through the tibia. Once the bone is cut, the top of the tibia which was initially angulated, is then rotated so that it's oriented in a level position. In this position the femur no longer slides backward, thus the knee is stabilized. A level tibial plateau essentially eliminates the physical need for the CCL. Metal plates and bone screws secure the cut part of the bone making it a strong repair.

CORA Based Leveling Osteotomy (CBLO)

CBLO is a newer procedure that is used to treat canine cruciate ligament disease. Like TPLO and TTA, a saw is used to cut through the tibia, but at a different location. The TPLO bone cut is at the uppermost corner of the tibia while the CBLO cut is lower down, sparing unfused growth plates in very young dogs. If your dog's surgeon recommends this procedure, be sure to ask how many times he/she has performed it and what the typical complications are. CBLO hasn't been tested by time and repetition compared to other procedures, so there isn't ample evidence of its long-term consequences. Because of its newness, CBLO techniques are still being refined. A compression screw was first added to augment the fixation. A more recently reported improvement was the addition of a position screw/pin and a tension band. These were incorporated because with the differential cut of the tibia, the pull of the quadriceps muscles can be strong enough to cause the tibial plateau angle (TPA) to shift. If you choose CBLO, please be sure that your doctor has been trained to use the latest enhancements.

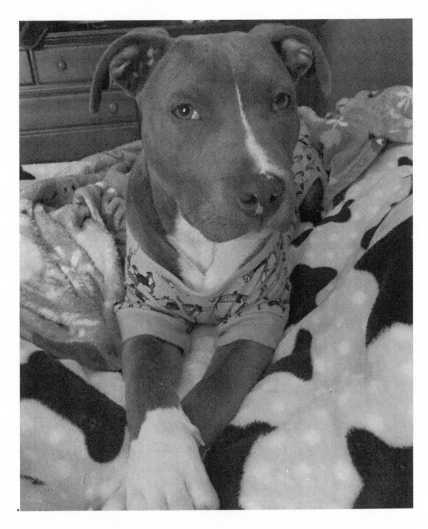

Two Crucial Consultations

A word of advice: You might read online accounts of people warning you to not allow too many veterinarians to examine your dog's knee because they'll cause further damage when they do the Cranial Drawer Test. This maneuver checks for excessive movement in the knee joint which suggests but is not definitive of CCL tear.

Some people say that after being examined their dog limps more, and this was the case for Vinny because he had two consults. Do I regret having him checked by two doctors and then being sore afterward? Not at all.

Think of it this way. If you needed a major orthopedic surgery on your knee, you'd see one doctor and then you might wisely get a second opinion.

Both doctors would do an orthopedic examination to assess how your knee moves. The integrity of your ACL would be checked using an orthopedic test called the Anterior Drawer Test. It's precisely the same movement the veterinarian does to your dog's knee with the Cranial Drawer Test. Orthopedic tests, whether for pets or humans, are designed to stress certain anatomical areas to help doctors discern which structure is injured and causing pain or dysfunction.

If a couple doctors did these tests to you, you'd likely limp back to your car in more pain than before you walked into the office.

To recap, some people who are against CCL surgery say that veterinarian orthopedic testing causes further injury and increased pain. If you want the most accurate diagnosis, the doctor must do a full examination.

For Vinny's initial surgical consult, I was referred to a vet who performed two lateral suture surgeries on their 40-pound dog, Chloe.

My friends also began with conservative management. They took Chloe to physical therapy which included exercises with a physical therapist, walking on an underwater treadmill (hydrotherapy) and getting acupuncture. Therapies helped, but not for long. After not seeing long lasting benefits, they decided that surgery was necessary. Chloe's surgery allowed her to joyfully run and play again. I wanted that for my dog, too.

The doctor examined Vinny and did an excellent job of educating me on how the lateral suture surgery is performed. She thoroughly answered all of my questions. I felt confident in her knowledge and ability. She doesn't do TTA or TPLO procedures.

She assured me that although Vinny was a muscular and active dog she felt comfortable performing this procedure on him. I thought Vinny might be too heavy as lateral suture is best for lighter weight dogs, so I asked about it. She explained that she's performed lateral suture repair on dogs heavier and more active than mine. And with 20 years of surgical experience, she felt confident that Vinny was a good candidate.

She checked both of Vinny's knees and said both CCLs were torn. Both patellae (knee caps) luxated which means the tendon that keeps the knee cap aligned slipped in and out of the groove in the femur. This also a source of pain. She recommended performing surgery on the left knee first, since that was the side he initially tore.

It was recommended that I consult with a vet who performs TPLO and recommended Board Certified specialist, Dr. Catherine Popovitch. I appreciated that she suggested a referral.

I scheduled with Dr. Popovitch who examined Vinny and said that with his size, strength and high activity level the TPLO would offer the most reliable repair. She prefers TPLO for large, muscular, energetic dogs.

Dr. Popovitch explained the critical differences between lateral suture and TPLO. Both procedures require the same post-surgery restrictions. The dog is not allowed to run, jump or be off-leash outdoors for a period of 12-weeks after surgery. When inside the house the dog should be kept calm and not be allowed to run, jump or go up or down lots of stairs.

The main difference with TPLO is that your dog can bear weight on the surgical side sooner because a metal plate and bone screws firmly hold the repaired area together. Metal is stronger than the cable used for the lateral suture repair and is why TPLO is a stronger fix. She confidently stated that she didn't recommend anything besides TPLO for Vinny.

After examining him, she agreed with the diagnosis of bilateral CCL tears. By this point, I had restricted running and jumping and he had worn the left leg brace for a while. Of the two knees, the one that had a more significant amount of scar tissue formation was the left side.

Remember that scar tissue acts to stabilize the joint internally. The right CCL was the newly injured side and unlikely to have much scar tissue formation at all. As a result, Dr. Popovitch recommended doing the surgery on Vinny's acutely torn right side. It made sense.

I read many accounts where people said they felt that doctors recommended the most expensive option because they wanted to make more money. However, I never felt that either surgeon made recommendations based on monetary gain.

I needed time to consider the options. I scheduled one more consult with Vinny's primary care vet, Dr. Warren. I described what I learned from both surgical consults, and he agreed that TPLO was the better option.

I scheduled the TPLO with Dr. Popovitch. I felt good knowing that I had done my due diligence for Vinny. We were finally ready to take on the next challenges.

Before moving on, let's take a look at surgeon credentials.

"Board Certified" veterinarians are accredited by the American College of Veterinary Surgeons (DACVS). They're the best of the best when it comes to knowledge and surgical expertise. Not only have they completed four years of veterinary medical schooling, but they've undergone an additional four years of advanced medical and surgical training. They have access to state-of-the-art facilities, equipment and support staff. For these reasons, their consultation and surgery costs are higher.

Non Board Certified veterinarians also perform CCL surgeries. Their consult and surgery costs are less than that of Boarded vets. If you choose a non-Boarded surgeon, ask how many hours it took them to earn certification to perform

the CCL procedure they're recommending. Ask h
times they've performed the procedure and wha
surgical complication rates are like.

While I understand the desire for primary care vets to grow their practices, expand their knowledge base and perform complex surgeries (versus referring out to Board-Certified surgeons), I believe that my decision to choose a Board Certified surgeon was the wisest one I made on behalf of my dog.

Here is an excerpt from a study pertaining to CCL surgical complications, published in 2007 by Lafaver et al: "Some of the major complications seemingly resulted from technical mistakes during the initial learning curve...We believe that they were technical failures related to surgeon inexperience. Attention to detail of the surgical technique cannot be over-emphasized and could eliminate these issues." The takeaway here is to choose a Board Certified surgeon based on their higher degree of expertise and experience.

Please do your research. Some doctors who aren't Board Certified offer a heavily discounted surgical cost to compete with more experienced surgeons, but understand that the discount could come with a great deal of surgical inexperience.

To find a Board Certified veterinary surgeon near you please visit this site: https://www.acvs.org/what-is-a-veterinary-surgeon.

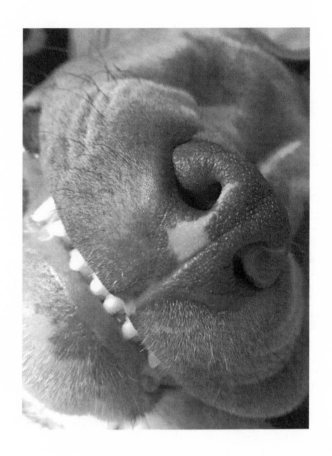

52

The Importance of Taking Notes

I wrote down lots of questions in a spiral notebook. It's easy to forget the timeline of things, especially when you're stressed and have such important decisions to make. Bring the notebook with you to every veterinary visit, and take notes. This keeps things organized and everything in one place. It makes it simple to go back to see what you did, to read about pain levels or other symptoms, to check when you gave meds or to re-read the doctor's answer to a question you asked.

When it's time to pick your dog up from the hospital, you'll be excited, anxious and stressed. We all know what happens to our memory when we're stressed. Bring your notebook along because you'll get so much information that by the time you get home you might forget crucial details. If it's written, it decreases worry as well as your odds of making mistakes.

The most valuable note taking will take place after surgery. Every time I gave a medication, I jotted down the time of day, which pill he was given and how many pills he got. I took notes about his appetite. I listed foods he ate and the ones he refused. I wrote what times I let him out to urinate, and I always wrote when he pooped. I kept track of times he seemed like he was in pain. I wrote down every symptom. And I noted my subjective experience for him – what it seemed like he was feeling and why.

You'll be so focused and absorbed in caring for your dog that one day will run into the next. You'll want to avoid thinking things like "Did I give the antibiotic today, or was that last night?" I relied heavily on the notes to keep myself organized.

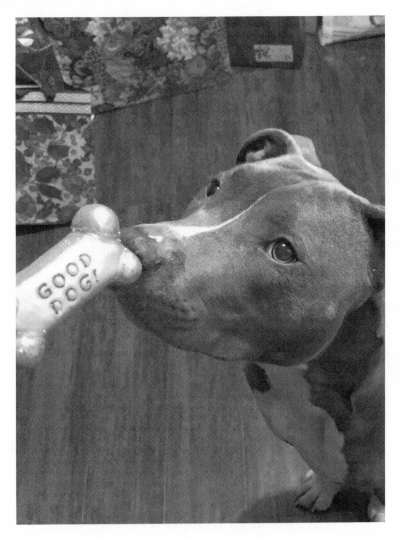

Should I Bathe my Dog Before Surgery?

There are situations where the surgeon might prefer that you bathe your dog beforehand. Many surgeons don't want us bathing our dogs for six to eight weeks post-op. They don't want the dog slipping, jumping or running. You know how dogs get the zoomies after they get bathed! So, in this case it's better to have spa day for your pup before surgery.

Another case worth bathing your pet before surgery is when they have skin conditions such as allergies that warrant more frequent bathing. In this situation, you should bathe him before surgery day.

I chose to not bathe Vinny before surgery for one main reason. No matter which shampoo I use, he gets itchy. He's just a sensitive little guy. I figured the post-operative discomfort was enough for him to deal with. I didn't want to add itchiness to the mix.

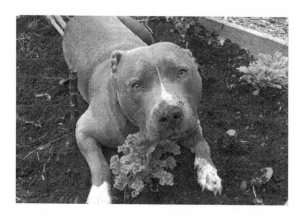

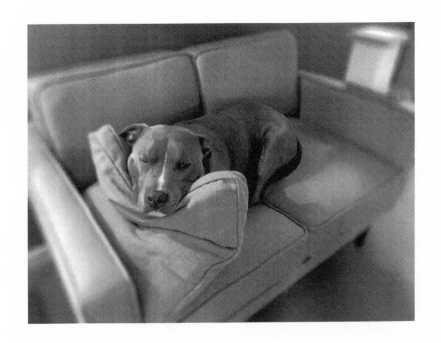

Surgery Day Is Here

Vinny needed to fast the night before surgery which meant no food after 8 P.M. and no water after midnight. That morning I felt sorry for him because he wanted his usual routine, which is to go outside and come in for breakfast. Sorry, little buddy!

We needed to be to the veterinary hospital between 7 – 8 A.M. When we arrived, they took him in and began prep. They put in his IV, sedated him and took specific X-rays for the TPLO procedure. Since he was getting an epidural they shaved a little square patch on his lower back near his tail. They also shaved the fur on his right leg all the way up to his hip.

It was the first time I ever left Vinny for such a complicated procedure. I never had him stay in a kennel or without me overnight. I worried about him being confined a cage. I expressed this to the nurse. She explained that being in a cage is a good thing after surgery because the dog is still sedated and not moving or processing things correctly. For that reason, being confined keeps them safe and prevents them from moving in ways that could cause injury.

If your dog is staying at the veterinary hospital overnight, please be sure that there is surgical staff is present 24/7. Surprisingly, some places don't have this. If trained professionals won't be present, I recommend that you ask to pick your dog up after surgery and take him home that day.

When the nurse took Vinny back for prep, he happily went along with his tail wagging. I felt confident that I made the best choice of all the options given, but I was still nervous about how it would all turn out.

A couple hours later I received a call from Dr. Popovitch saying that everything went well. Thank goodness! She dealt with the luxating patella issue. Both menisci were intact and didn't need repair. She saw mild arthritis, which I expected.

Later that day and into the night I called a few times to check on Vinny. The nurses said his pain was well controlled. They had to wait a while for the anesthesia to wear off before he was interested in getting up to urinate. He wasn't interested in eating the kibble they offered, but at dinnertime he ate some boiled chicken.

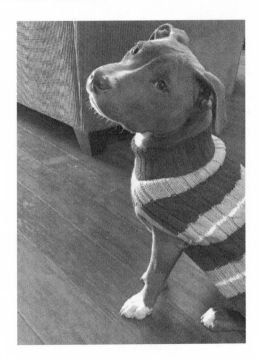

Prepare Your House Before Your Dog Comes Home

While Vinny was recovering in the hospital, I was busy cleaning and prepping the house for his arrival.

You know how it is when you're sick and all you want is peace and quiet? Set up his recuperation area in a quiet spot away from main entry doors or where there's commotion. I set up his recovery spot in the living room so he could be close to me, and I could keep an eye on him.

Although he loves laying on the couch that faces the back yard, I didn't want him to jump on it, I slid the sofa to another room. In its place went a futon mattress. I put half of it against the floor atop a 5x5 piece of rubbery non-slip material and the other half went against the wall. It was a ground-level comfy place for him to rest and heal.

The futon mattress was a better option than buying him a bigger dog bed. He generally lays stretched out in a straight line rather than curled up in a circle, so the futon mattress was more than long enough to allow him to do that. I washed the futon cover and all of his blankets so that everything that came into contact with his leg was clean. I used laundry soap without fragrance and didn't use scented dryer sheets.

If your house has slippery floors, you can lay down unrolled yoga mats or throw rugs that have rubber backing so they won't slide when stepped on. These will greatly improve traction. Make sure the edges of rugs or yoga mats aren't curled up because you might trip over them yourself.

Although a crate was recommended for Vinny's recuperation, he hadn't been in one for years. When I tried crate training him as a puppy he hated it. There was no reason to stress him out or risk having him get hurt by trying to escape it after surgery.

I had an exercise pen from when he was a puppy. It's a series of panels that attach to one another. I used it to keep him in the living room and to restrict him from running from one room to another. I put the gate up in an arc around the front of his futon mattress.

As his mobility improved, I used a couple exercise pen panels to restrict him to whatever room he chose to be in. He did fine this way and showed no interest in running, jumping or trying to knock the panels down.

The exercise pen panels can easily be knocked down or fall over. If your dog is nervous in a crate or if he suffers from separation anxiety and you worry about him knocking down ex-pen panels, ask the surgeon about getting meds such as Trazadone to keep him calm while confined.

Remove all opportunities for your dog to jump or access stairs. I read many stories where people came home after CCL surgery to find their dog not where they left him. Either he was upstairs, downstairs or lying on the sofa or bed. These are common culprits for surgical setbacks.

Even though there's a metal plate and screws holding the bone together (with TPLO, CBLO, MMP and TTA) or a strong synthetic cord that's been woven from one bone to the next (lateral suture and tightrope), the surgical site has a certain degree of fragility until it fully heals. One jump could be all it takes to reverse what the surgeon did.

Simple ways to reduce the risk of jumping include:

• Putting up gates to keep him away from steps and furniture
• Tilting couch cushions so he's blocked from jumping up
• Closing bedroom doors to prevent jumping on beds

For your safety, be conscious of the baby gates or exercise pen panels that are around you. Avoid falling over one yourself. Use nightlights so you can more easily see gates or other barriers at night.

My bed is one of Vinny's favorite spots to lay on a sunny day. To thwart his desire to jump on it I made a major modification. I took the mattress off the box spring and put it directly on the floor. I disassembled the headboard and took it and the box spring to the basement. For a time, no more headboard, no box spring and just the mattress. Ugly? Yes. Safe for my dog? Absolutely. Vinny loved it, and when he transitioned from wanting to sleep on the futon to sleeping on the bed, we both slept soundly.

There's more about the sleeping situation in the chapter, "Good Night Sleep Tight".

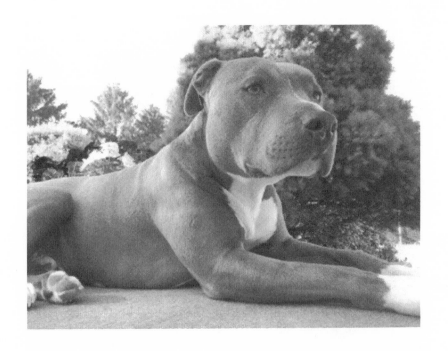

Housekeeping to do Before Your Dog Comes Home

Prepare the area where he'll spend most of his time. Before I thought of how best to care for my dog, I imagined the way I like things when I'm not feeling well.

With all of the cleaning you'll be doing, here's a tip you might not have thought of. Dogs have a sense of smell that is markedly more powerful than that of humans. Whatever you smell, your dog smells it more than you do because he literally has several million more scent receptors than you do.

You'll clean, wash and dry clothes, maybe burn a candle, and you'll think everything smells so fresh. But when your dog comes home, he'll be in pain and possibly nauseous from medications and anesthesia.

Imagine a time when you were in a lot of pain or were extremely nauseous. Think of how awful it would be to walk into a room that reeked of your grandmother's stinky, flowery perfume. Yuck! When we aren't feeling well the last thing we want is to smell strong scents, right? It's why I highly recommend that you use as many unscented products as possible, especially after he comes home from the hospital. You should skip diffusing essential oils for the same reason.

I made sure I got everything done before Vinny came home. I washed the futon mattress cover and got it back on the futon. I dusted, swept, moved furniture, vacuumed and mopped.

Have clean blankets ready to keep him cozy after surgery.

After a couple days of him being home, you could set up an area outside for him to enjoy a change of scenery. Lay down a blanket or sheet to protect the incision from contacting the ground. No matter how perfect the weather is, lay a lightweight blanket, sheet or pillowcase over the incision to protect it from exposure to direct sunlight, dirt and insects. A heavy blanket will weigh-down his leg, so opt for something lighter.

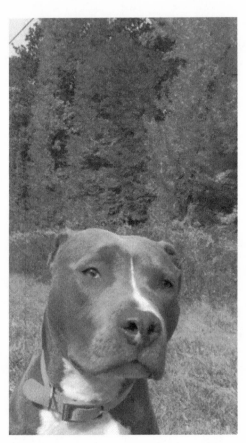

It's Time to Bring Your Dog Home

Have your car packed with these things before you pick your dog up from the hospital:

- Blanket or comforter to cover the back seat
- Pillows or blankets to fill in the gap of the floor to make it level with the seat (gives big dogs a larger area in which to lay)
- Harness/Sling (or bath towel if you didn't buy a harness)
- Leash with collar attached
- Your spiral notebook that has questions for the doctor written in it
- Your list of *"Ask the Expert"* discharge questions (discussed in this chapter.)

Before they bring your dog to you, you'll get discharge instructions from the surgeon, nurse or vet tech. You'll get lots of information, so if there are two of you, one should be the listener and one should take notes. To avoid missing something in the notes, ask the veterinary staff person if it's okay to record the conversation using your cell phone or other recording device. Practice recording and saving a conversation using your phone's voice memo before the discharge appointment. I've recorded things and inadvertently deleted them many times.

You'll learn about medications and the dos and don'ts of caring for your pet. There's a blog post on RunAgainRover.com that has a comprehensive list of questions to ask at discharge titled, *Ask the Expert*. You should print it and bring it with you. Too many people leave the discharge appointment never asking some of the most basic of questions.

Besides asking the right questions, I highly recommend asking to see your dog's before *and* after X-rays. This needs to be done by a doctor, so it would be wise to request this ahead of time.

Familiarize yourself beforehand as to what X-rays look like for the type of procedure your dog had. Seeing the X-rays isn't enough; use your cellphone to take pictures of each X-ray view. First, look for your dog's name on the corner of the radiographs. You'll want to see that your pup's plate or implant and screws are intact. Are the screws are protruding more than a few millimeters from the other side of the bone and into the muscle? If so, ask the doctor about it. Ask to be shown areas where there's evidence of osteoarthritis. And the most important question of all: Is there any evidence of post-op fracture? Have them show you an intact post-op tibia and fibula. You must know that there aren't any fractures *before* taking your dog home.

We've all gotten teary-eyed watching videos of people being reunited with their pets. I watched one where a man picked up his dog after surgery. He sat on the floor and his Golden Retriever sat quietly with him, one paw on each of the guy's shoulders as though the he was getting hugged. Although it was sweet and anyone would love to have the same response, don't gear yourself up for anything like that.

You'll be thrilled to see your dog and excited to bring him back home away from all of the noises, smells and people he's not used to. You'll hope for bionic-butt tail wagging when he sets eyes on you. Not so fast. Things went down a lot differently when I picked up Vinny.

As the nurses brought him out from the back and were slowly walking him toward me I quietly said his name. "Hi, Vinny." I hardly got a reaction. I wasn't sure he recognized me. He slowly limped to me wearing the plastic e- collar. The techs encouraged him to walk, but he was still feeling the effects of the anesthesia and medications.

There was no tail wagging or doggie hugs. But I didn't care. I had my baby back, and the next phase of our journey together was about to begin – healing.

I previously put down a folded blanket across the entire back seat. I filled in the gap between the floor and the car seat with pillows to create a larger base on which he could lay. I extended the blanket forward to also cover the pillows.

Rather than having fluffy blankets or a comforter, I recommend keeping the surface where he'll lay as flat as you can. This makes getting him out of the car easier because his leg won't catch on bunched up material. Have a friend or family member go with you when you pick up your dog so they can sit by his side as you drive. If your dog is large, I highly recommend having a helper.

If your pup is groggy when you pick him up from the hospital, he'll need help getting out of the car and might need some assistance to remain standing. Guide him by holding his sides so he doesn't fall. Or you could use a beach towel as a sling. If you purchased a harness, it might be tricky to put it on him, especially if he's groggy.

Some dogs aren't groggy, and those are the ones who are so happy to be home that they jump out of the car and run. Surprisingly, this isn't uncommon. Be ready! Have your pup's collar and leash on and held securely before you open your car door. If you're going to get him out of the other side of the car, close the car door before you walk around to the other side. Don't assume that he's incapable of jumping out and running away.

See whether he's interested in a potty break before you take him inside. Chances are that he didn't sleep well the night before, so it would be good for him to pee first so that when he's settled inside he can get a long nap.

He's been given IV fluids, so he might need to pee. If he's sniffing around, be patient because it might take a bit longer than usual for him to urinate. Because he fasted before surgery and likely hasn't eaten much afterward, don't expect him to poop. If he tries lying down, it's because he's groggy or in pain. I recommend not letting him lie outside at this point and getting him into the house instead.

Once he's inside, get him to his designated area. Encourage children to play and talk quietly. I kept the TV and radio off. I did quiet things, such as reading, computer work, cooking, sweeping or washing dishes. I avoided using loud household items such as the vacuum cleaner or dishwasher. I remind you of this because it keeps the space calm, which is how humans prefer things when we don't feel well. I think our dogs want that too.

Vinny was so content when he got home. He was back with his kitty brothers and sister. He smelled the usual smells and heard the usual sounds. I'm sure on some level that was comforting. He slept so hard that he snored.

Some people wonder whether it's okay to leave a dog in a dog run or secured in a yard. This is unwise. A perfect weather forecast doesn't change this. What seems to be an ideal outdoor arrangement isn't safe enough without supervision. After a week or two, you might think he's well enough to be alone outside, but there are far too many factors that you can't control.

Weather is unpredictable. What if your dog got tangled in the leash or whatever you used to tether him? What would happen if a stray, injured or sick animal came into contact with him? What if a stranger approached your dog? He could chase squirrels, birds or other animals. If he moved abruptly, ran too fast, jumped or fell this could lead to unnecessary pain and suffering for your dog. It could result in an emergency veterinary visit or worse, an additional surgery. The safest place for recuperation is inside your house. He should be monitored at all times while outside.

This is important: Make or print a sign to cover your doorbell or on hang any door where visitors or delivery people frequent. The sign should read, "Do not knock or ring bell! Dog recovering from surgery." This helps reactive dogs to remain calm during their recovery. Hang signs on doors inside the house reminding family members to have the dog's collar and leash on before the door opens. I have printable signs like these ready-made and available in my Facebook group. Have you requested to join yet? We're waiting to meet you and your pup, so don't forget to check us out!

Here's the link: www.facebook.com/groups/CCLsurgery/

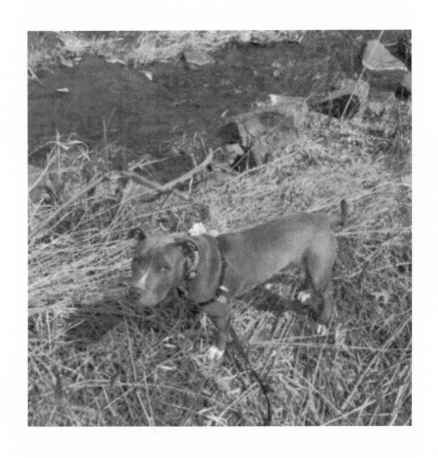

Should You Stay Home from Work or Get Help?

I'm a small business owner with a flexible schedule, so I was fortunate to be able to be home with my dog the first week after surgery. I scheduled surgery on a Thursday so I could pick him up and stay home with him Friday through the weekend and the following week.

With a complex procedures like these, it's my feeling that someone should be with him for at least the first week after surgery. If you can't do that, I recommend asking a neighbor, friend or relative to stay with him. If you know you'll need outside help, look for pet sitters who have experience caring for post-op pups. Your dog's primary care vet might have recommendations. You'll feel a lot better knowing someone is there to watch over or check on your pet. Think about how it is when you're not feeling well. Isn't it nice knowing someone is nearby?

Let's revisit the dog watcher app I eluded to in an earlier chapter. There are several to choose from in the app store. You'll need two devices. Each needs to be connected to Wi-Fi. You'll point one smartphone or tablet with its camera focused on your dog, and the other smartphone or tablet stays with you. Some apps allow you to hear your pet and talk to him.

There are also affordable cameras available on Amazon. Some don't require a Wi-Fi connection. Regarding apps and cameras: I wouldn't have felt comfortable using either of them to monitor my dog during the crucial first-week post-op (unless I worked close by and could get home quickly if something required my attention). I think they're best for short-term monitoring during times when pet owners or caregivers need to step away for a moment.

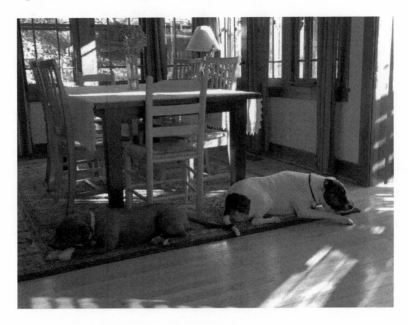

Harnesses and Slings

Before I picked Vinny up from the hospital, the nurse recommended assessing his ability to walk before I decided whether or not to get a harness. She mentioned commercial under-the-belly types as well as trying a folded-up towel as an under the belly sling. IMPORTANT: If your dog is having a bilateral procedure, I absolutely recommend getting a sling; do not use the "wait and see" approach with bilateral pups.

I recommend trying a towel sling before surgery day to assess whether you can physically manage it. This might take a few attempts, so don't give up prematurely. Do multiple practice sessions per day inside your house as there are less sight, sound and smell distractions there. Once you're successful, practice outdoors.

No matter which type of sling you use, practicing weeks to a month before surgery creates muscle memory for you and your dog. You'll have it properly sized and you'll know how to apply and remove it. Your dog will become familiar with the way it feels on his body as you assist and walk by his side.

The towel method didn't work for us because I found it awkward to use and couldn't maintain a strong grasp on it because my dog is heavy and it kept slipping out of my hand. I had to hunch over as we walked, which aggravated my middle and lower back. If you suffer from chronic back pain or sciatica, I don't recommend using a towel sling, especially if you have a large breed dog.

The towel sling was also challenging because I had to manage too many things at once – keeping myself balanced as I moved, effectively supporting my dog's weight and then having to make sure he was steady enough to let go of the towel so he wouldn't urinate on it. For male dogs you can try shifting the towel forward the moment before he goes to urinate, but this is nearly impossible. Or you could let go of the towel before he urinates, but you need to be sure he's able to stand on his own and that by letting go of the towel that he doesn't fall.

When using a sling, don't lift your dog's hind legs off the ground because it puts pressure on the spine and shoulders. Think of it this way: Remember being kids when we walked on our hands as another person walked behind us grasping our ankles? Imagine the feeling in your back, arms and shoulders if the person lifted your legs too high off the ground. Your job with the harness is to pull upward with enough force to assist walking while still allowing his back paws to contact the ground. It's actually beneficial for him to put some weight on the surgical side. When using a harness, you'll need to provide more lifting support at first and then less as he heals. If your dog is a male, don't be surprised if he lifts the non-surgical side to pee and puts full weight on the repaired side. You don't need to control this if it happens.

The Gingerlead® harness is a popular choice among dog owners, veterinarians and canine physiotherapists. Both harness handles fasten together with Velcro, allowing for firm grip and control. If harness parts become soiled, it's machine washable. It's adjustable for height so you can stand straight while assisting your dog. It's made in the USA.

Some inexpensive brands are made of flimsy material that gathers up under the dog's belly. Gingerlead® uses a soft, plush material that holds its shape and doesn't bunch-up. This is surely more comfortable for your pet.

If you have a male dog, certain harnesses cover the dog's penis. Some males will refuse to urinate if the harness is creating pressure near their anatomy. You can slide the sling forward just before he urinates then slide it back to allow for easier walking. A mistake that people make in an effort to keep the sling away from the dog's penis is by positioning the material too far forward on the dog's body. This creates a force of pull that's directed from the belly rather than at their hind end, the area we're most interested in lifting. Gingerlead® has a specially shaped sling that doesn't get in the way of their anatomy and allows them to urinate freely (it can also be used for females). They also offer a rectangular-shaped sling that's made for females.

I've seen instances where some dog owners lose grip on harnesses or towel slings, and once the dog realizes they're free, they take off running! Gingerlead® has this covered. Attached to the handle is an adjustable length leash, allowing you to maintain control and the ability to walk the dog with one hand.

The Gingerlead® leash can attach to an optional chest harness. This feature is helpful for older dogs who also need support under the front of the body and/or support as they go down stairs. When our dogs become seniors, this can be a useful add-on feature if they need walking assistance.

Unlike Gingerlead®, some harness brands have lots of straps and clasps making them difficult to fit and then remove. The solution for some people is to leave it on their pet 24/7. This can't feel good for the animal, especially because one of the straps rubs wraps around the shaved surgical hind leg near or against the incision. There are images online of dogs who suffered from painful skin ulcerations and chafing.

Another well-known brand is The Help 'Em Up Harness. I can't stress the importance of this enough: I highly recommend watching the fitting instruction video on their website before your dog comes home from having surgery to be sure it fits properly. You'll want adjust the straps ahead of time and be familiar with using it well in advance of surgery day because trying to size this harness for the first time on a post-op dog will surely be a painful experience for you and your pet.

There are two types of Help 'Em Up harnesses available for male dogs. If you're unsure as to whether yours will need a special attachment so the brace won't cover his penis, there's a video on the company's site that you should watch. As you view your dog from the side, if his penis is visible the regular harness will work just fine. If it's located farther back and hidden between his hind legs, you'll need the brace with the special attachment. The company reps say that most dogs don't need this attachment.

Another standout feature is that it has two handles, one at the level of the shoulders and another farther back toward the hind end. This distribution evens out the force of the pull making it more manageable for you and likely more comfortable for your dog. The best part is that this type of harness offers a lot of support without putting excessive upward pressure on the dog's abdomen or spine.

Unlike other brands, the Help 'Em Up can be used by two people at once for heavy dogs. Someone holds the front handle while the other holds the back. I found that the direction of pull is more evenly balanced if one person stands on the dog's left side and the other person grasps the handle from the right. If both people stand on the same side, the direction of pull comes from one direction and pulls the dog in that same direction making it difficult to walk in a straight line. I'll admit – it's awkward with two people, so this recommendation is primarily directed to people who have very heavy dogs.

The hind leg straps have a padded sleeve which I feel is inadequate because it still caused redness and irritation on the sensitive skin along my dog's inner thighs, especially on the surgical side that was shaved. Fabric stores sell a soft material that resembles lamb's wool. Purchase a couple small pieces. Sew a tube that's long enough to fit over the hind leg harness strap/s. Placing it on top of the padded sleeve coverings will provide added protection and comfort. You could do this for both hind leg straps or just for the surgical side. I recommend making the sleeve and using it *before* any skin irritation starts.

Putting the Help 'Em Up Harness on your dog can be made easier by marking the fasteners and hooks. Connect the harness straps as though it's on your dog. Wrap pieces of masking tape or electrical tape around each hook and strap. Use a permanent marker to label where each piece connects with a corresponding number. The next time you put the harness on your dog will be easier because you'll know to attach the hook of strap "1" to the fastener marked "1".

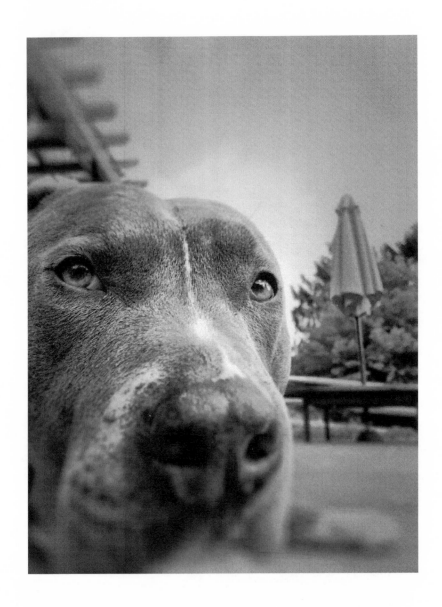

The Incision Site

Before he has surgery, peruse some online images of what your dog's leg will look like afterward. Notice the amount of swelling and bruising. Look at the incision length and the way the sutures or staples appear. Look for the reddened areas which might not only be bruising, but razor burn from being shaved for the procedure.

Seeing these things beforehand will help you to more effectively monitor the healing process. Some people take day-by-day pictures to track the healing process. Pay attention to those because it will give you something by which to compare your dog's results. If you're squeamish about medical stuff, some preparedness will help you to not be shocked or grossed out by what you'll see.

The post-op images I saw online of other dogs showed much more swelling than Vinny had. His swelling and bruising were mild with both procedures. His surgeon applied a compression bandage post-surgery, which helps to control swelling. It was removed before I brought him home. The surgical nurse told me that not all doctors do that, so it would be wise to ask your dog's surgeon beforehand.

Vinny's surgeon did three layers of sutures. The two deeper layers dissolve on their own and don't need to be removed. The outermost layer was removed two weeks post-op.

The removal process didn't seem painful. The worst

part was trying to hold him still. If your dog is anxious when going to the vet's office, an anti-anxiety medication such as Trazodone could be helpful. Talk to the veterinarian about anti-anxiety meds at the time of his first surgical consult. I'll review medications in a separate chapter.

After the stitches were removed Vinny's incision was perfectly straight. All but the very top of it was flat. I palpated a pea-sized swelling there. There was no redness or oozing and it wasn't hot to the touch (these are signs of infection). The doctor said it could be a reaction to the dissolvable stitches that were underneath and that it will flatten day by day, which it did. There was also a sesame seed sized dot under the skin's surface at the very top of the incision. That's where the suture is knotted.

Bruising will become evident quickly, but a day or so post-op is when reddened areas that look like brush-burns appear. This is due to razor-burn from the leg being shaved. Some veterinarians recommend putting a thin layer of Vitamin E oil or a thin layer of Triple Antibiotic cream over it to soother the chafed skin. Before you do either, check with the doctor or nursing staff.

Some surgeons send dogs home wearing a bandage over the incision. They'll advise you when to remove it. Removal can be difficult because the adhesive clings so tightly to the skin. If you can't easily remove it, don't rip it off quickly despite what you've read online. Why put your dog through more pain? Don't chance ripping off layers of skin (this sometimes happens when people rip bandages off). A little time and patience goes a long way.

You can use these things to remove excess bandage glue or the bandage itself: coconut oil, vegetable oil or olive oil. Dab it on with a cotton ball, Q-Tip or tissue. These oils naturally soften and loosen adhesive without irritating the already sensitive skin.

Warning: There is bad advice online as to the use of toxic chemicals and other household items to remove bandage adhesive.

These irritating products include things such as: vinegar, peroxide, nail polish remover, engine starter fluid (someone in a Facebook support group for CCL recovery actually suggested this), rubbing alcohol and Goo-Gone. Each of these is caustic, potentially toxic or irritating to sensitive skin and should be avoided.

Do not apply anything to the incision unless the surgeon recommends it. You shouldn't clean the incision with irritating things such as hydrogen peroxide or alcohol. If you take him outside and mud or dirt gets on the incision, gently dab it off using a soft cloth moistened with warm water. Then gently blot the area dry with a soft cloth. If you feel the area isn't looking good or that it's not healing well, call the veterinarian right away.

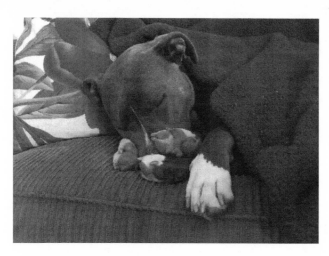

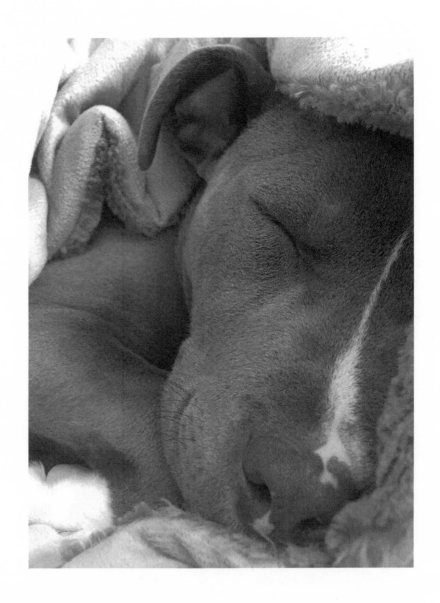

Good Night, Sleep Tight

I read stories of how people had awful nights trying to sleep next to their dog. People set up sleeping bags or a row of couch cushions next to their dog's bed. Many gave into the fact that there would be a lot of sleepless nights.

Here's where the bed solution comes in. This only works if your bedroom is on the first floor. It won't leave your bedroom looking suitable for a Pottery Barn catalog, but you'll have a better chance at actually getting some much needed shut-eye.

I mentioned this previously: You could remove your bed from the frame and put your mattress directly on the floor. Move the headboard, frame and box spring out of the room. Don't leave the box spring under the mattress because your dog might try to jump onto or off the bed. Even the low height of the box spring and mattress together is still too high of a jump.

With just your mattress on the floor, you and your dog will sleep better than trying to get comfy on couch cushions, an air mattress or in a sleeping bag. Just like when a child is sick and feels comfort by sleeping next to a parent, your dog will feel cozy and calm with you nearby. With him sleeping by your side, you'll be able to monitor pain, if he needs to go outside, or if he attempts to lick the incision.

My dog woke up every morning after surgery around 1:00 A.M. needing to urinate. For this reason, the first three or four nights after surgery, I slept on the futon mattress I had set up in the living room, which is near the patio door to the backyard.

During the day the futon was in an "L" shape with half on the floor and the other half against the wall. I pulled it away from the wall before bedtime so it was flat against the floor. If you don't have a futon, you could try a mattress topper with some blankets above or underneath to make it comfier.

Your dog might suddenly need to urinate for many reasons: from being given IV fluids during surgery, a medication side-effect, increased water drinking or merely waiting until last minute because moving hurts. It can be difficult getting your dog to the door where he'll go outside. This is why for the first four or five nights we slept on the futon which was only steps away from the door that leads to the yard.

When you're woozy from sleeping it can be tricky getting the dog outside. Have everything lined up and ready to go. You don't want to have to do any thinking. Keep things where they're easily accessed. It's wise to have a night light to avoid trips and falls.

Make it a habit before you go to bed to set up everything you'll need to let him outside: have his collar already attached to the leash. Have the harness/sling (or towel) nearby. Have a raincoat or other jacket next to the door. Take a flashlight with you if there isn't a light outdoors. Put Kleenex in your pocket before going out in case he has diarrhea and needs to be wiped. Have your shoes ready, with the left one on the left side and the right on the right side. Vinny wanted to go out in the middle of the night. I was so groggy. I got his harness and collar on. My coat was on, and I stuck my feet into my boots so quickly that I had them on the wrong feet. At that point, he was whining because he had to pee. I didn't have time to fix the situation, so off we went, both of us hobbling around the yard! You can bet that every night thereafter, I set my boots up so all I needed to do was slip my feet in and go.

After a couple weeks he wanted to be in the first-floor bedroom, which is where he usually sleeps. Rather than to buy him a cushier dog bed, and instead of having him sleep with me and getting kicked all night long, I got him a narrow twin memory foam mattress from Amazon. I put it on the floor alongside my mattress.

Vinny prefers to lay on his side with his legs straight out, which was true especially after surgery. He's not a dog that sleeps curled up in a circular-shaped bed. This is why it didn't make sense to put his dog bed next to mine. Getting him the mattress bought both of us a more restful night's sleep. He still chooses to sleep on it.

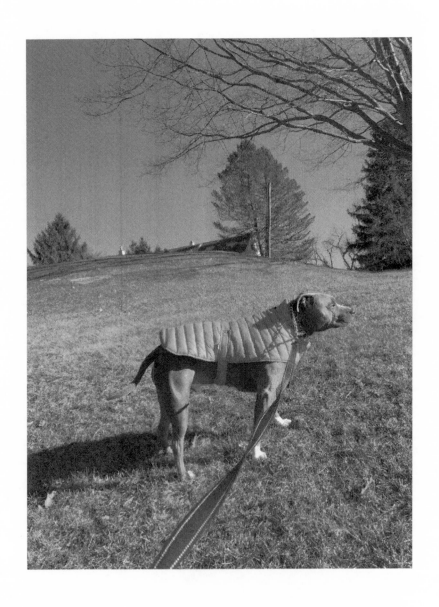

The Importance of the Cone Collar

Dogs hate them. They scrape against the walls and ground. They cut off their visual field of view. Wearing it while resting or sleeping is cumbersome.

If your dog tries licking his incision, without question it must be worn. If your dog will be alone after surgery, it's safest to use the conventional cone collar they had on him when you picked him up after surgery. And whatever you do, even if you purchased a soft material or inflatable e-collar, don't throw away or recycle the plastic one your dog was sent home wearing. You might end up needing it down the line.

With any e-collar, make sure he's unable to reach the incision while wearing it. Observe him wearing it for a while before you assess whether it works or not.

A word of caution about any non-plastic e-collar. Vinny wore an inflatable one for less than ten minutes before he managed to wedge his front paw through the neck hole. It's not a big deal if you're there to catch it happening, but imagine what could've happened if he was alone when his leg got stuck! If you use an inflatable one, it's intended to be worn with the regular collar threaded through the loops along the inside of it.

When I was there to supervise, I removed the e-collar so he could rest with his head flat down. Sutures can be damaged quickly if the collar is off and you get distracted by other pets, children, household chores, phone calls, etc. Be especially aware of your dog during these times. If you need to step away, make sure the e-collar is on.

I remember the nurse's reminder when I picked Vinny up from surgery. She said, "Whatever you do, don't let him lick the incision site." When it comes to nighttime and sleeping, if you sleep like a rock it's best to make him wear the e-collar at night to be sure he doesn't lick the incision. You have to weigh the benefits versus risks when you choose the collar (inflatable versus cone-shaped).

He won't feel comfortable wearing the plastic "cone of shame", but if you're a sound sleeper, and he licks the incision or bites at the sutures, you could have a situation where the sutured skin tears apart (wound dehiscence) or becomes infected.

When I spoke with a doctor about post-surgical infections, she said that the dogs that licked the incision a lot are the ones most likely to have complications. Licking introduces bacteria into the incision. This could cause a terrible infection of the bone called osteomyelitis. A skin infection called MSRP (Methicillin-Resistant Staphylococcus-Pseudintermedius) could also occur; both infections can cause serious complications.

What to Do When He Gets Antsy

The doctor said it was okay if he lays on the surgical side. In doing so, he's able to put the majority of his weight onto the non-surgical hind leg to go from lying to standing. I was told it was okay if he stretched out on his belly with his legs straight out behind him. No matter what position your dog chooses, he'll eventually become sore and will want to move. I recommend assisting him until you can see he's able to manage on his own. Sometimes it takes only a few days for him to figure it all out.

If he needs help, simply scoop your hands under his butt to help him switch positions or to go from lying to standing. Be careful of the stitches and his sore knee. Be sure you're lifting correctly by bending at your knees. If there are loose blankets around him, move them out of the way so they don't catch his paw or leg on the side where the incision is. Slowly lift his bottom as you say, "Up". Initially, it will be awkward to move him, but he'll eventually catch on and allow you to help.

To give him a change of scenery, I put his dog bed on the deck. Sunshine, fresh air, and experiencing the outdoor sights, sounds and smells were so good for him. He was leashed with me by his side the entire time to keep an eye on him. Lay something light over the incision to prevent exposure to the elements, dirt and insects.

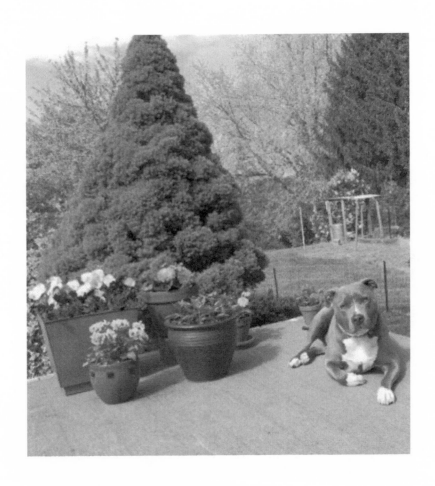

Taking Your Dog Outside

Because he fasted before surgery and likely hasn't eaten much afterward, don't expect him to poop for up to four days after surgery. As days progress and he's eating close to normal amounts of food, if he's still not having a bowel movement, contact the veterinary hospital.

Just as you would typically do, gauge the frequency at which you take him out based on how much he's eating and drinking. Regarding urination - a reminder that he was given IV fluids in the veterinary hospital to keep him hydrated. Even if your dog isn't drinking much water, you'll still need to take him outside because of the fluids. Medications could cause increased thirst, which results in increased urination.

Sometimes your dog will whimper, cry, quiver or seem restless. These could be signs that he's in pain. It could also mean that he's anxious, but before you jump to give him anti-anxiety meds consider taking him outside. You know how uncomfortable you sometimes feel when you need to go to the bathroom? His body is no different.

If he's feeling pain, he could seem disinterested if you ask him to go outside. If he can't get up on his own, and it has been a while since his last potty break, try scooping your hands under his bottom and slowly lifting him as you say, "Up". If he doesn't electively walk, this still might not mean that he doesn't need to urinate or defecate. After he pees or poops he'll likely come in and settle down nicely. Remember the signs he showed you before you took him out so you'll recognize them if they arise later on.

If you didn't purchase a harness, manually support under each side of his butt as he squats. This was awkward for me and made my back hurt. The harness made it so much easier for both of us. Peeing is physically easier for your dog, but pooping requires an even-balanced squat and some pushing with the back legs, which could cause pain. Giving him some verbal reassurance as he poops the first few times.

For the first few weeks when I let Vinny out to urinate he peed much longer than usual. I was letting him out more frequently and thought that doing so would help, but no matter how often he went out still he still did marathon pees. Many times, he chose to stand on the side that was surgically repaired. After he stopped taking all of the medications, the urine volume and frequency returned to normal.

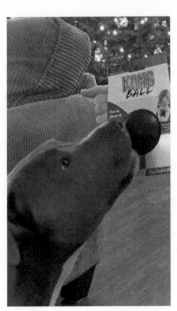

How to Help Him Eat

Bringing Vinny's food and water bowls to him for the first week made it easier. I put down a dish towel and slightly tilted his bowls toward him. This worked out well and allowed me to save the times that he was up and moving for when he needed to go outside to do his business.

Your pet will eat and perhaps drink less than usual for a couple of days after surgery. Assume this will occur and don't force him to do either. His appetite will return to normal once a few things happen: the anesthesia clears from his system, pain becomes well-controlled and after he begins moving around more frequently. Notify the vet if he's not interested in eating for more than a day or so.

Pain medications often cause constipation. Have a can of 100% pure pumpkin on hand. This helps to hydrate the dog and soften stools. Pumpkin adds bulk to stools in the case of diarrhea. All it takes is a small amount of pumpkin to do the trick. Ask your veterinarian how much to feed based on your dog's weight.

Get some good quality canned dog food. I started with a couple cans of chunky style and some of the smooth pâté type Wet food can stimulate his appetite if he becomes disinterested in whatever you typically feed him. Either mix in some of the canned stuff with his dry food or use it in place of kibble. You can hide his pills inside of little meatballs that you make from pâté style canned food. It's more hydrated than kibble and may help to avoid constipation. You'll need something that he's willing to eat when he takes pills that are to be given with a meal, so having extra food options on-hand will make things less stressful for you down the line.

Buy some chicken meat and rice. This is an excellent option for a dog who refuses to eat dry kibble or canned food.

Plain yogurt without vanilla or sweeteners of any kind will give your dog protein and gut-friendly yogurt culture to help with diarrhea.

Purchase some creamy peanut butter. I use the natural kind without sugar. This is a handy way to hide pills. Peanut butter is high in fat, which could cause diarrhea and also irritate the pancreas, so don't give your dog excessive amounts.

Buy eggs. When my dog got fussy with food choices there were times he ate a couple scrambled eggs. Be sure to allow them to cool down before offering them to your pet. You could hard-boil eggs as well.

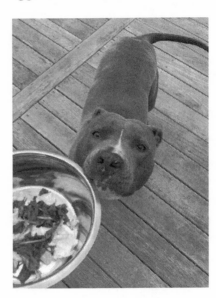

Medication

Medications cost more when we get them from veterinarians. Sure, we can leave the office or surgical center with the meds our dogs need, but we're paying a hefty markup for that convenience. If you know the names of the drugs your dog needs, go to www.GoodRx.com to compare drug prices at pharmacies near you. Simply ask your dog's primary care vet or surgeon to fill the prescription wherever the best deal is. Easy!

Ask the surgeon or nurse about how often they gave pain meds to your dog. I recommend that you continue their dosing schedule when you bring your dog home. I gave the pain meds their way consistently for just over a week.

Another question to ask is which pills can and cannot be crushed. Pills are bitter tasting, but some people say the only way they can successfully get their dogs to take them is to crush them and put them into food that the dog loves. Before doing this, make sure the doctor says it's okay because some medications have special coatings that are meant to dissolve slowly once in the animal's body.

When your pet is able to move around more easily, ask the vet whether you should decrease the dosage of the pain med at the time intervals listed on the pill bottle or if you should lengthen the time between dosages and give the same dosage as is listed on the pill bottle. Ask when it's safe to discontinue giving pain medication.

Pets experiencing pain can feel nervous and anxious. If anxiety continues, it could heighten pain symptoms. I asked the doctor whether having a sedative on hand would be helpful. She said it isn't necessary for all dogs, but for ones that are high strung or nervous, a sedative such as Trazodone could be used. Wanting to be prepared, I had a prescription for the sedative filled, and I'm glad I did.

The first couple nights after surgery, he was quite antsy and having a hard time settling. He wasn't crying, but he couldn't get comfortable. I stayed by his side to soothe him so he'd feel safe and calm. For the first week post-op, I gave him the sedative before bedtime. It helped him relax and get quality sleep.

Trazodone should be administered one to two hours before you need it to do its job. So, if you plan to go to bed at 9:00 P.M., give the sedative between 7:00 and 8:00 P.M. When you administer the dosage, jot down how long it took to become effective. Knowing this allows you to strategically administer it the next time he needs it. Giving it on an empty stomach might increase its efficacy, but it could also cause stomach upset.

Sometimes I worried that Trazodone would overly sedate him, so I gave a lesser dosage. Not surprisingly, it was ineffective. Get help from the veterinary staff if you have dosage questions about any medication.

Before surgery, Vinny was prescribed Deramaxx. It's an anti-inflammatory drug. His primary vet prescribed it when he tore his CCL the first time. It helped him walk without as much pain and limping. Rimadyl, Metacam and Previcox are other common anti-inflammatory medications.

IMPORTANT: NSAID medications increase bleeding, so if your dog is taking an anti-inflammatory, ask the surgeon well in advance of surgery day when you should stop giving the medication. Dr. Popovitch asked that I discontinue administering Vinny the Deramaxx one week before surgery.

Before Vinny was fitted for the stifle brace he was taking Deramaxx. He took the medication for the prescribed two-weeks after which time he needed blood work to make sure it wasn't affecting his liver or kidneys. If his levels were normal they'd prescribe more. By that time, he was limping less, which I attributed to his wearing the brace I elected to wait on having the blood work done because I wasn't sure he needed another refill.

Looking back, I see this was nothing more than wishful thinking. The longer the time without Deramaxx and the more he wore the brace, the more he limped. I went ahead and brought him in for the blood work. His liver and kidney values were within normal range, and we restarted the medication. Once again, I noticed a vast decrease in his limping. I'll address this medication again in the "My Mistakes" section.

Some medications cause side effects including but not limited to the following:

- loss of appetite
- nausea
- nervousness
- muscle twitching (fasciculations)
- pacing
- tremors
- vomiting

If your dog exhibits any questionable reaction to medication or if he develops an atypical symptom or behavior, get a video of it, place a phone call to the veterinary team and send the video to them to get their advice about what to do next.

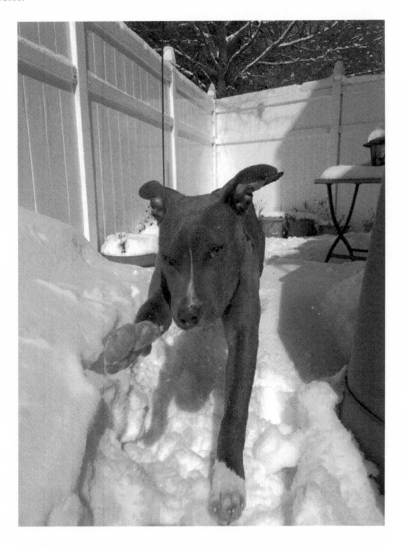

Dealing with Antibiotic Side-Effects

After surgery, antibiotics are necessary because they prevent bacteria growth which can lead to infection. During surgery, your dog was given IV antibiotics. Some surgeons prescribe them prophylactically and others do not. Ask the surgeon whether your pet will need them post-op.

If they're prescribed, stay on track with the dosages. If you miss a dosage or you're concerned about side-effects, contact a professional at the surgical center for advice.

Sometimes antibiotics cause side effects. Every animal has beneficial bacteria that regulate proper functioning of the digestive system. Gut bacteria is also known as gut flora. Antibiotics kill off nasty bacteria that cause infections, but they also kill the beneficial ones that regulate the gastrointestinal (GI) system.

The GI system goes from mouth to anus and is comprised of the stomach, intestines and colon. When the GI tract flora is balanced, bowel movements are neither too hard nor too soft. Antibiotics disrupt the balance, so bowel movement consistency and smell might be different from what you're used to seeing.

There's a possibility your dog could have regular bowel movements for the first few days of taking antibiotics then diarrhea could begin later on. This doesn't mean you should discontinue giving the antibiotics. If your dog is nauseous, vomiting or has diarrhea, call the veterinary hospital and let the experts advise you as to how to proceed.

Giving antibiotics with a full meal can reduce tummy upset (follow label instructions on the pill bottle). Plain yogurt helps too. Remember - plain yogurt is without vanilla flavoring, sugar, artificial sweeteners, or fruit. Sugar feeds bacteria, so give the plain, unsweetened kind.

At the time of Vinny's first TPLO surgery, he weighed just over 70 pounds; I usually gave him about 1/4 cup of plain yogurt, sometimes less. If you're unsure of how much to feed, ask the vet.

Vinny tolerated antibiotics for a week with minimal side effects. A few days after surgery he was eating normal amounts. Then a significant shift happened. After a week or so, his stools turned from normal-loose to outright diarrhea. He wasn't as interested in eating, and infrequently he dry-heaved. I called the veterinary hospital. They recommended Pepcid and asked me to continue giving the same dosage of the antibiotic. Pepcid alleviated the stomach upset and dry-heaving.

The Pepcid dosage depends on your dog's weight. Call the vet's office to get proper information. Check with a doctor first, and don't self-medicate.

Remember that I mentioned canned pumpkin for diarrhea? When a dog has diarrhea, canned pumpkin bulks up the stool making it firmer. There's an important distinction; canned pumpkin and canned pumpkin pie filling are not the same. Pumpkin pie filling has sugar and spices in it. Look for pure canned pumpkin with no other ingredients. If all you have is pumpkin pie filling, wait until someone can go to the store to get pure canned pumpkin. Don't go overboard by giving too much of it for a couple of reasons. Think about how you feel when you have a stomach bug or how you might feel after having surgery. The last thing you'd want to do is eat a lot of anything, right? Well, your dog is the same.

Pumpkin is high in Vitamin A, which in high amounts can be toxic to dogs. Give a teaspoon or two for a small dog, and maybe a couple tablespoons for a larger one. Again, ask the veterinary staff about how much to feed if you're unsure.

Avoid giving fatty foods and table scraps. Fatty foods cause diarrhea. If your dog already has looser than normal stools or diarrhea from the medications, it would be wise to avoid giving him fatty table scraps.

If medications or stomach upset makes your pet picky or disinterested in eating his usual kibble or canned food, offer boiled chicken (skin should be removed) mixed with a little white rice. You could add a bit of pumpkin to the mixture. Diarrhea can lead to dehydration, so adding some of the broth from the boiled the chicken will help with that. You could also add meat broth, meat stock or bone broth, but look for brands without onions and garlic, which are toxic to dogs.

If your dog loves chicken and rice and gulps it down, watch out, he could vomit. Instead, give smaller amounts of food at a time. You can control the speed of eating by hand-feeding him. If you usually feed your dog 1 cup of kibble, offer the same amount of chicken and rice. It's better to offer him 1/2 cup twice with 15 minutes between feedings than having him vomit after gulping down the entire cup. Always offer fresh water after he's eaten solid foods.

Is your dog allergic to chicken? Use turkey, pork, bison or venison because these are lean meats. Fatty meats are more likely to cause diarrhea and include fattier cuts of beef, veal, duck and lamb. It doesn't mean they can't be used, but decrease the meat portion with fattier cuts. Scrambled or hard-boiled eggs are a good source of protein and other nutrients.

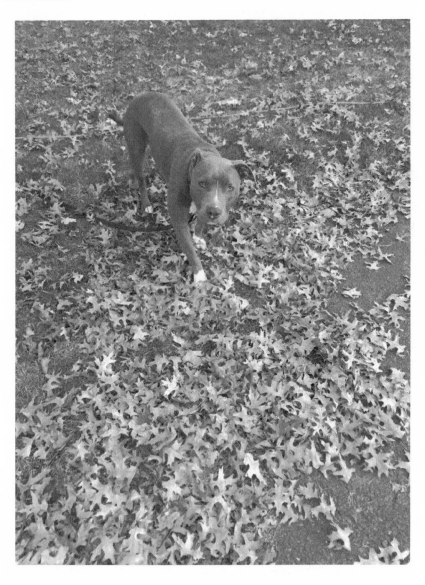

How to Know When Your Dog is in Pain

Animals in pain can show some or all of these signs:

- Panting or breathing with the mouth open (if it's hot outside or inside your house, don't necessarily excuse panting with the temperature)
- Shivering or shaking
- Whimpering or crying out
- Biting or snapping

If you've stayed on track with giving pain medications and you see any of the symptoms listed above, notify the surgeon and her staff ASAP.

When humans are given medications to control pain, doctors and nurses say, "It's important to stay ahead of the pain." That means that we don't want to take the medication and then allow for so much time to lapse before taking the next dosage that the pain level shoots up to an excruciating level.

Think about it this way: Consider pain on a zero to ten scale where zero means no pain and ten is pain that's so unbearable that you need to go to the emergency room. A 10/10 pain level is an excruciating, uncontrollable pain – the worst pain you've ever experienced.

Let's consider a pain scenario to give perspective regarding "staying ahead of the pain". Say your pain level a half hour after taking pain medication is a 3/10. You take the next dosage when the label recommends, which is eight hours later. Your pain increased to 4 or 5 out of 10. That's what we want. The pain level only slightly increased. Here's where it goes wrong.

You might say, "My pain is only 4/10, I can handle that, so rather than to take the next dosage when I'm supposed to, I'll wait a few more hours." Instead of taking the med in eight hours you take it in eleven hours. By that time the pain has risen to 9/10. You're suffering at that point, and taking the medication after the pain has gotten that high makes it more difficult to control. When the medication finally kicks in, your pain might only reduce to a 7/10. That's still a lot of pain. Do you understand what I mean?

You didn't stay "ahead of the pain". Staying ahead means staying on time with the dosing schedule and not allowing the pain to get to an uncontrollable level.

Some people are anti-medication and want to wean dogs off the meds sooner than prescribed. Consider this, the humane thing is to use the medication to help your dog feel his best. If he's in terrible pain he won't be able to get up to go outside. He might not want to get up to eat or he could lose his appetite altogether. He will likely have difficulty getting restful sleep, which is when the best healing takes place. Uncontrolled pain isn't beneficial for optimal healing and recovery. Give pain meds as directed by the surgeon. Assess him after a couple days, and see whether you can or should alter the dosing (with guidance from the staff at the veterinary hospital).

Even though your dog is getting meds to control pain, he'll still be sore, especially when it's almost time for the next dosage.

For this reason, and I mentioned this previously, I recommend bringing food and water bowls to your pet for the first week. Hold the bowls low enough and slightly tilt them toward your dog so he can easily eat while he's lying down. Right after he eats, offer him his water bowl so he can have a good drink of fresh water. Allow for extra time in the morning to get the dog fed, let outside and settled. Understand that morning time and before bed can be challenging, as pain levels can be more pronounced at those times.

The body heals during sleep. Controlling pain at bedtime is essential. Over time you could slowly adjust the time of day so that he's given the pain med an hour before bedtime. It will help him (and you) sleep more soundly. Get help with the timing of giving meds by talking to the veterinarian and his/her staff.

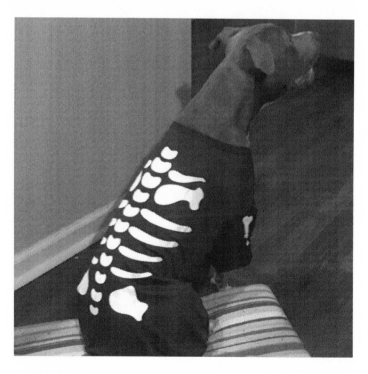

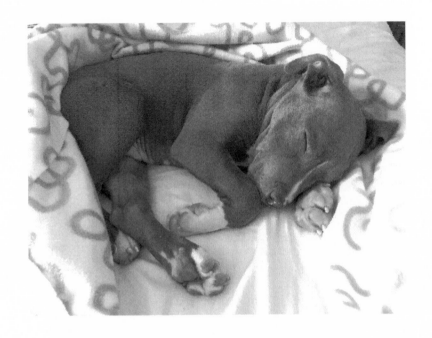

Normal & Abnormal Signs at the Incision Site

These are typical occurrences during the healing process:

- Bruising of the leg around the upper, mid and lower leg
- Swelling of the leg at the level of the incision and down to the paw three or four days after surgery
- A minor amount of clear or blood-tinged discharge coming from the incision site
- Warmth of the leg on which surgery was performed
- Discomfort at the incision site
- Redness or swelling of the skin around the sutures
- Redness of the skin due to razor burn

These are abnormal incision signs. Call the surgical center at once if you notice any of these:

- Oozing pus or blood from the incision site
- Extreme redness at the incision site
- Large amounts of discharge coming from the incision site
- Swelling that doesn't decrease in three to four days
- An incision that appears to be opening
- A red bump that appears along or outside of the incision area

Another issue that can occur is a seroma. A seroma is a fluid-filled pocket that occurs near the incision site. Some describe it as feeling like a jiggly water balloon and others say it feels mushy rather than firm.

Seromas are common in post-op dogs that physically overexerted during the early phases of recovery. The fluid inside rarely contains white blood cells, the presence of which suggests infection. If you see a fluid-filled pocket developing near the incision, take a pictures and videos each day to monitor. Some surgeons suggest warm compresses, while others recommend leaving it alone, so ask your doctor about which treatment they prefer. Your dog's body will eventually resorb this fluid and the swelling will reduce. Draining seromas isn't always necessary because when punctured, what was likely a sterile pocket of fluid could allow bacteria to enter through the needle puncture site and result in an infection.

IMPORTANT: If you see anything questionable regarding the incision, take pictures and videos each day to monitor. Ask ahead of time for a veterinary team member's cell phone number so you can send the images and get advice ASAP.

Dogs often have problems on weekends or after hours. Be sure to get a cell phone number during the surgical discharge appointment so you can get expert advice when the veterinary hospital is closed.

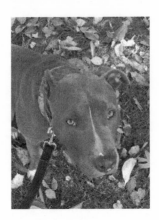

Managing Boredom

The way you and your dog are used to interacting and playing will change after surgery. You'll need ways to manage his boredom. There are online videos showing fun games you can play while he's lying down. There are Facebook groups dedicated to canine enrichment.

I purchased natural white marrow bones from my local pet store. They're plain and not coated or filled with any type of flavoring. I filled the hollow center of each bone with a grain-free canned dog food and froze them. It was a nice treat for Vinny to concentrate on for about 20-minutes. You might have to wait until his appetite is back to normal before he's interested in these. Some people make mixtures of different things to fill bones including: plain yogurt, kibble, peanut butter, apple sauce and bits of veggies or cheese. Too much peanut butter and fat in general can inflame the pancreas (pancreatitis), so be aware of not going overboard with fat.

Changing up the scenery is a great way to manage boredom. I put his dog bed on the deck in a sunny spot to let him get fresh air and be stimulated by the outdoors. I covered him with a blanket and always made sure the incision site wasn't exposed to the elements or direct sun. Keep him on-leash so he can't run or jump. Bring a book or your computer outside and sit with him. Being outside will be a nice change of scenery for you, too!

When you've been told he's allowed short walks, keep them close to home. It's wise to limit them to your driveway, the sidewalk near your house or in the yard itself. Walking the neighborhood leaves you and your dog vulnerable to approaching dogs, friendly or not. Minimize putting your pup in environments where he'll be tempted to jump, run or lunge. This includes places where there are lots of people, birds, squirrels and other animals. If you have another pet that's playful and might interfere with his walking, I recommend exercising them separately.

For the first month or so it's not wise to put your dog in the car to go walking somewhere, even if it's a place he loves. For that reason, I don't recommend dog parks, walking trails, or open areas. It's best to be in an area where the surroundings are relatively predictable. Keep it simple and safe for him for the first month.

I recommend walking on a flat surface. His knee won't do well if he has to walk over stones, sticks, twigs, branches or ruts in the grass. Maintain a relatively straight walking path and avoid having him make sharp turns.

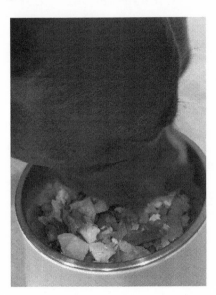

Post-Surgical PT at a Facility or at Home?

This book isn't meant to guide you through daily at-home physical therapy because there's already plenty of information in books and online, but I'll share with you what I did.

No matter what you've read so far about conservative or post-op therapy, keep in mind that each dog heals differently. What one dog is able to do at a certain timeframe might be very different than what another dog can do. Don't rush things.

Let your dog guide you with the exercises. If he's struggling, don't force him to do therapy. If he's resisting, try some encouragement, but if he continues to resist, let it go and end the session. If the dog is licking, shaking, panting or snapping at you, you should obviously skip the exercises that day. If limping increases, end the session and revisit PT another day.

There is a good post-operative home rehabilitation guide that recommends doing passive range of motion (PROM) on the surgical side right after surgery. Passively bending and straightening my dog's leg was difficult because the swollen skin was so tight. The leg straightening (extension) was easy, and Vinny didn't mind it. He didn't like the flexion (bending) part. I think it stretched the sutured skin too much, and I hardly flexed the knee. The last thing I wanted to do was pull the skin apart or break stitches, so I stopped doing it, even though the exercise manual recommended it. I restarted

PROM after the sutures were removed, and he allowed the it without resistance. You must use your own discretion when it comes to physical therapy. Doing exercises based on a generalized timeline isn't appropriate for every dog.

At every stage post-op, my boy loved massage. I always supported under his knee with one hand and massaged with the other. I massaged his back legs, shoulders, back, neck, chest and front legs. Don't put direct pressure on the incision.

A couple days after surgery, I warmed his leg before the massage by saturating a washcloth in hot water, thoroughly wringing it out and laying it flat inside of a Ziploc bag. I pushed the air out of the bag and sealed it. Tap water is hot enough for this. Don't put the washcloth in boiling water because it will be much too hot and can burn your pet. Before applying it to your dog's leg, test the temperature by applying it to the inside of your forearm.

He enjoyed lying on his heated dog mat, so sometimes I had him do that before the massage. We took short walks, as recommended by his doctors and nurses. After our walks I applied ice using a sealed bag of frozen peas or a small icepack atop a dishtowel. Don't use the hard, plastic-coated ice packs or heavy ice packs that could weigh-down the leg.

As the duration of his walks became longer, if I was supposed to walk him for 20 minutes and saw him limping at 15 minutes, the walk ended. I made up the time later with another shorter walk. I wanted to keep him exercising as pain-free as possible, which is how PT is done for humans, too. The no pain, no gain type of exercising is an old-fashioned way that creates more trouble than it does good.

You might have read online that you can make icepacks by filling a Ziploc bag with a mixture of rubbing alcohol and water. I don't recommend this because we all know how those bags leak. If you've ever scraped or injured your skin and applied alcohol to it, you know how it makes an awful stinging sensation. The last thing you'd want is for a homemade icepack to leak alcohol on your dog's sensitive incision. Either buy a couple bags of frozen peas or purchase a couple small, icepacks. Always place a thin towel between your dog's leg and the ice pack.

Puppy squats (wall sits) are recommended in a popular home rehab guide during the early phase of healing. I didn't like the idea of forcing my dog's knee to flex so much when he was still swollen and before his sutures were removed. I'm glad I waited because I read an online review where a woman explained that her dog popped his stitches open after doing puppy squats too soon. This is called wound dehiscence, which is painful, causes setbacks in healing and requires a visit to the surgical center to be re-stitched.

After the stitches were removed I retried the wall squats. I stopped doing them because Vinny was physically unable to sit comfortably with either leg squarely under his body the way most dogs do.

I asked a veterinarian about this at a follow-up appointment, and he said some dogs can sit normally after surgery and some never will. Mine is the latter. I don't believe in forcing him to sit in a way that looks better but causes him pain. While the puppy squat exercise might be beneficial for some dogs, it didn't help mine, which is why that exercise got nixed early on.

We did figure 8's with wide turns around two kettlebells that I set up inside. You can use anything: gallon jugs of water, laundry detergent containers, bricks, or anything that your pup isn't inclined to play with. You could do these outside as long as the ground isn't mushy, snowy, icy or bumpy. If the ground isn't flat I would do the exercises inside. Bumpy ground will stress the knee joint.

In general, lousy weather makes joints hurt more, so exercise indoors in inclement weather. Except for two small steps to access the grass I didn't allow Vinny to go up or down stairs in the house. I followed the surgeon's instructions to not allow him to run, jump or go off leash for 12 weeks.

At his final follow up appointment, I asked whether having him do underwater treadmill therapy or PT at a veterinary PT center was recommended. The doctor said it's best for dogs who are showing a lot of muscle atrophy at eight to twelve weeks post-op. He said that dogs who avoid using the leg a month after surgery are the ones who need PT done at a facility. He looked at Vinny and said he was healing very well and that we could continue doing exercises at home.

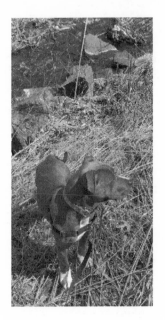

My Mistakes

The majority of the mistakes I made happened before surgery. Here are things I shouldn't have done:

Hoping the pain and limping would go away on its own:

When I watched him sit and walk strangely I hoped it was a transient symptom that would resolve on its own. When a dog has persisting symptoms, even if they seem to last a short time or if the symptom intermittently comes and goes it's a sign that something is wrong and warrants veterinary attention.

Allowing him to go outside off leash when he first started showing signs that his knee was injured:

Dogs with torn CCLs can still run and jump, so don't let that fool you into thinking he's okay. They shouldn't be allowed to do either because further damage can be done to the CCL. Any helpful stabilizing scar tissue that has formed is weak and can be easily broken down.

Feeling sorry for him and letting him occasionally run to chase a squirrel or bird because it's what he loves to do: (see previous answer)

Being tricked by a pain-free day:

If he was having a relatively pain-free day I thought that his perhaps his knee was healing. This was far from the truth because he'd look fine one day and be lame the next.

Not ordering replacement straps for his brace as soon as I got it:

It took too many days to get the replacements via postal mail, which meant I wasn't adhering to the wearing schedule the way I was supposed to.

Deciding to stop giving his anti-inflammatory meds on my own:

Allowing him to be off Deramaxx for a couple weeks because I thought the brace was helping and that he might not need the medication. It was foolish. Even if the brace was working, there was likely inflammation, which the medication could have controlled. Inflammation and pain decrease together. They go hand-in-hand.

Not giving his anti-anxiety medication correctly:

It should be administered one to two hours before sedation is needed. Your dog's weight determines the dosage. Giving a lesser dosage than was prescribed made it less effective.

Differences Between Left & Right TPLO's

Just to recap: My dog had bilateral (right and left side) CCL tears. TPLO #1 was done on the right side. TPLO#2 was done on the left side eight-months later.

Knowing whether surgery was necessary or not:

Before the first TPLO, I was unaware that surgery was imminent. Understandably, I tried whatever I could to avoid it. There were joint supplements and natural anti-inflammatories, cold-laser treatments, physical therapy exercises, a custom-made brace, range of motion exercises and massage. Perhaps at best, it gave us some time, but any positive results were short-lived.

Having been through TPLO surgery less than one year prior, when he re-injured the opposite leg, I knew enough of the signs and symptoms to say, "This is more than a little tweak." Deramaxx wasn't working, which made me think it was more serious than a transient inflammation. He was three-legged-lame the entire time, even with the meds. The only conservative measures I took the second time around were daily massages to his legs, back, neck and chest to counter the muscular compensation and extra pressure being placed on other joints because of the limping. I scheduled surgery after a two-week trial with Deramaxx.

How he acted when I picked him up from the hospital:

The day after his first surgery when I picked him up

from the hospital, he was so groggy that it was difficult getting him into and out of the car. He had a tough time walking out of the hospital because he was still quite sedated. It seemed like he didn't know who I was. This is why I think it's important to have a helper come along. Try to find someone well in advance of the day you'll pick up your dog. You'll feel better knowing someone's there to assist.

With the second TPLO, when I picked him up from surgery he was much more alert. I still needed help getting him into and out of the car once we got home. Although he was semi-groggy, he visibly recognized me and seemed happy to see me.

Whether I needed a harness or not:

I had to rely on the Help 'Em Up Harness after his first TPLO. Remember, he had torn both CCL's. After surgery, not being able to bear immediate weight on the surgical side meant he had to put full weight on the left side. Since he had a torn CCL on that side as well, walking was painful. The harness was a must have.

After the second TPLO, he was able to bear all of his weight on the right leg, so I infrequently needed the harness. I'll keep it in case he needs it in his later years.

How long it took for him to use the leg after surgery:

Although he touched his paw (surgical side) to the ground a couple days post-op with the first surgery, I'm not sure it was because of some miraculous response to surgery. Even though I was using the harness, he physically had to use the right leg because the left CCL was injured and painful, too.

After the second procedure, I noticed that he took much longer to bear weight on the left side. This is because he could rely on the stronger right leg to hold him up. It took a full two weeks for him to touch the left paw to the ground, and even then, it was inconsistent. Up to five weeks after surgery, when he was outside and on walks he used the left leg, but whenever he stopped moving or when he stood still, he raised the left paw off the ground.

Waking up in the middle of the night to go outside:

I didn't notice excessive drinking after the first surgery, but he woke up several times during the night to go outside. His urine stream was more forceful than usual and it took longer than usual to empty his bladder. This could've been because he was given IV fluids in the veterinary hospital. Days after he came home the only thing I could blame it on was a medication side effect or that he was just so uncomfortable that he needed to get up and move.

With the second TPLO, he slept more soundly. There were nightly trips outside to pee for the first few days. The urine stream wasn't as forceful as it was after the first surgery. He wasn't whimpering to get outside like he did after the first TPLO. The Fentanyl patch (used with the second TPLO but not the first) could've been doing a better job of controlling pain. Perhaps I was better with the timing of dosing the Trazadone (anti-anxiety medication) and other medications. His response to the second surgery just seemed easier in general. I wonder if having been through it once before made it predictable in some way for Vinny.

Waking up in the middle of the night to re-situate himself:

With the first surgery, he was restless. He needed help shifting from one side to the other and to go from standing to lying or vice versa. I helped him do this several times a night.

After the second TPLO, he maneuvered himself around with greater ease. I believe it was due to improved pain control, which was likely due to the Fentanyl patch. Again, I believe his prior experience with TPLO recovery made the second procedure easier for both of us.

How long it took for him to have a bowel movement:

Everyone whose dog has been through one of these procedures knows how it is to become obsessed about when their dog will finally poop. I was no exception. It took three days after the first TPLO for that to happen.

I remember a quote I once heard from a nurse who said, "People can't expect to eat like birds and poop like elephants." It's true for people and pets! Your dog's appetite will decrease for a while, which means he'll poop less. He won't be physically active which will contribute to sluggish GI motility. Pain medications slow GI function, so that's another reason for the delay in the digestive system working as it usually does.

Remember to frequently offer your dog water. Vinny would not go to his water bowl to drink, but when I brought the bowl to him he'd lap it up. Offering low sodium chicken broth, bone broth without onions or garlic (toxic to dogs), veggies, fruits (no grapes because they're toxic to dogs) or canned dog food will maintain hydration so he'll have an easier time having a bowel movement.

On the day I picked him up from the second TPLO, we got out of the car, and he pooped right away. This was not a normal looking bowel movement. It had a slimy consistency and was an orangish brown color. It smelled much worse than usual. He pooped every day after surgery, but it took days for the color and consistency to return to normal.

Pain levels and whining:

After the first surgery, he whined quite often. This could be blamed on pain or the after effects of anesthesia. As he healed day-by-day, the crying related more to his wanting attention. I soothed him when he cried. If he was bored, I'd sit outside with him, I played enrichment games to stimulate his curiosity or gave him treats or a frozen food-filled bone to work on.

After the second TPLO, it was as though he understood what was happening. I was more efficient in my ability to care for him. As I previously wrote, pain and anxiety were managed better after having gone through surgery twice. Collectively, these factors made for a more contented, less whiney, less painful dog the second time around.

Appetite:

Vinny loves to eat. After the first surgery, it took him three days before he was interested in food. I tried his usual kibble (Nulo brand), and he only ate a few bites. Canned dog food didn't initially entice him. Scrambled eggs with a bit of cheddar cheese made him happy, and that was the first real meal he had post-op that he gobbled down.

After TPLO #2, there was a significant change in his appetite. Even the foods he usually loves were unappealing. This included his kibble, scrambled eggs, little pieces of cheese, canned dog food (I tried Zignature, Merrick and a couple other grain-free brands). I buy pâté style because it's easiest to stuff into the marrow bones that I freeze. So, I tried the chunky varieties of the brands I mentioned, and hooray! He liked them!

Because he wasn't overly interested in eating, giving meds that required food became tricky. I made little meatballs with the pâté style food, but since he didn't like it, I ended up having to pick the pill out of the food and then hide it in a little glob of peanut butter. Peanut butter always worked for giving pills. I tried cooked ground beef and ground chicken. I got one or two feedings out of them and then he refused it. That said, don't fry up huge portions of meat.

Stomach upset and diarrhea:

The antibiotics after the first TPLO were given until they started making him dry-heave and have consistent diarrhea. This began around the sixth day. I called the veterinary hospital after he had diarrhea a few times in a row. Canned pumpkin wasn't helping. Knowing that prolonged diarrhea leads to dehydration (among other things), I contacted the doctor. She recommended that I stop giving the antibiotic.

My strong recommendation is to get the doctor's advice before altering antibiotic dosages. Post-op infection can cause a myriad of serious complications, so for the sake of your pet's health, let the doctor decide what's best. Vinny needed Pepcid for stomach upset. The dosage is based on your pet's weight, so again, before administering it yourself, check with the doctor beforehand.

After the second TPLO, he wasn't interested in eating for almost four days. He'd eat a few bites and give up. I ended up buying a new brand of kibble because he refused to eat the kind I usually feed him. He liked the new kind, but not for long. I tried cooking chicken, ground beef, scrambled eggs...not a lot of interest in any of these. If he's not eating, try hand-feeding. You might be surprised at how well this works!

Much like after the first TPLO, he liked peanut butter and chunky canned dog food. Sometimes giving him the pill in a glob of peanut butter stimulated his appetite enough that he'd eat some food. Diarrhea began on day three. He vomited once, too. The doctor advised that I stop giving the antibiotic as well as the Rimadyl. At that point the Fentanyl patch was still on, so there was ample pain control. Stopping the oral medications made the diarrhea go away. After the Fentanyl patch was removed, I re-started the Rimadyl again, this time without noticing any adverse effects.

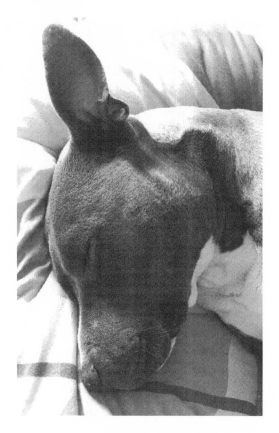

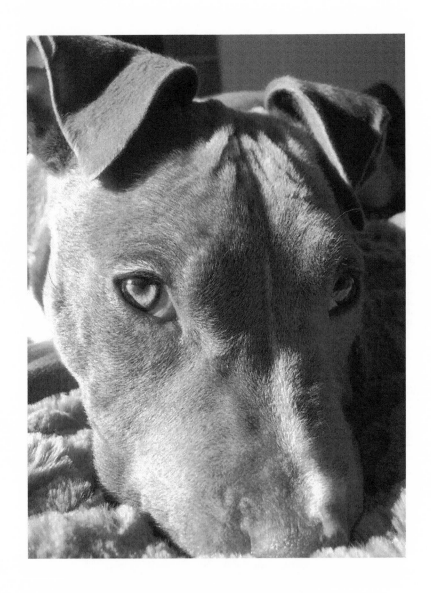

124

Products in My Amazon Affiliate Store

To see or purchase these items, visit my Amazon Affiliate store at www.RunAgainRover.com.

- Unscented Sardine & Anchovy Omega-3 Supplement (*CAN THIN BLOOD. ASK SURGEON WHEN TO STOP ADMINISTERING THIS IF YOU'RE SUPPLEMENTING PRE-OP)
- Heated dog mat (choose correct size online)
- Organic Turmeric Curcumin with Ginger & Boswellia
- Yucca extract
- Glycoflex Stage 3 supplement treats
- Gingerlead Harness (choose correct size online)
- Narrow twin memory foam mattress
- Exercise Pen
- Comfy Cone/Inflatable E-Collar (choose correct size online)
- Natural marrow bones
- Snuffle Mat
- DVD's for dogs
- Dog treats & toys
- Pepcid
- Heating pad
- Car/Stair ramp
- Lickimat
- Coconut oil
- Ice packs

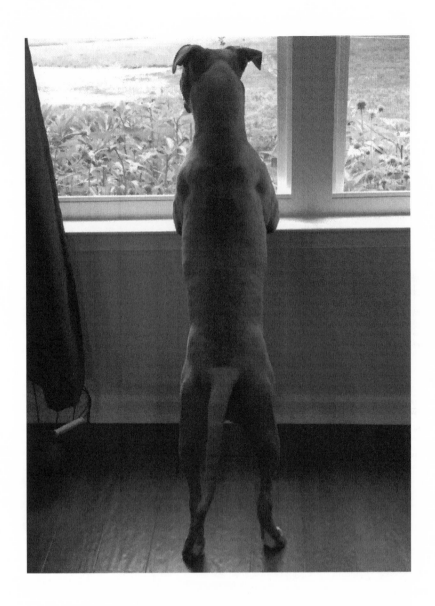

Best of Luck to You!

I hope this book was valuable to you. Be patient with the ups and downs of the recovery process. Most times you'll feel like you're doing an awesome job of caring for your dog, and then one little setback can make you feel disheartened. Whatever you do, hang in there.

Things will improve, and soon your dog will be running and enjoying things the way he always did. Don't be afraid to ask for help from the veterinary hospital staff where the surgery was performed. The people there are dedicated to helping you help your dog have an excellent recovery.

Best wishes for your dog's full recovery!

One Last Request

If you found this book useful, I'd be grateful if you took a few minutes to post a short review on Amazon.

Your support will encourage other pet owners to purchase the book and get prepared for what lies ahead. Please tell your pup's primary care veterinarian and the surgeon about this book. Educated and prepared pet parents make things better for surgeons, too!

Please type this into your web browser to post your review: https://amzn.to/2SbIYSH

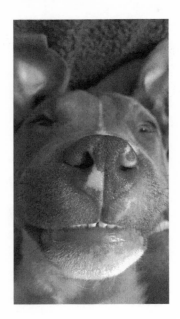

About the Author

Carla Spinelli is the proud owner of a pit bull named Vincent James. His CCL injuries began a journey of learning for both pet and pet owner worthy of sharing with others.

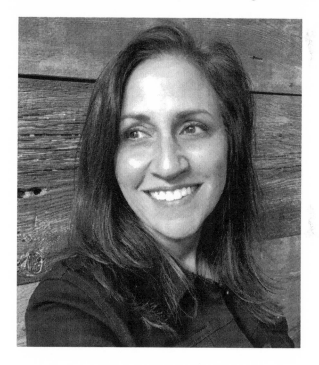

Made in United States
Orlando, FL
08 April 2022

16591497R00083